TRAINING LOG

for use with any elite level athletic training program

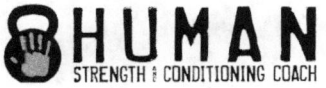

HUMAN
STRENGTH & CONDITIONING COACH

Developed by Duncan S. Sailors

CONTENTS

How to Use the BLOCK Annual Training Plan Tool

The BLOCK planning tool can be used to create an annual training plan. It is a tool to record any significant event or series of events that you are training for like a race or multiple races, a lifting meet, Regional or National Competition.

You would also want to include any significant event that would affect your training - Business trips, Holidays, Vacations, Medical events, etc.

IMPORTANT: Write in *pencil* - because plans change.

Guidelines:
- BLOCKS of training are broken down into CYCLES.
- BLOCKS can have any number of CYCLES.
- CYCLES can be anywhere from 1 week to 4 weeks long.
- You might think about a BLOCK as a season, with the CYCLES being the months in that season.
- Use letters for BLOCKS and numbers for CYCLES.
- BLOCKS and CYCLES are used throughout this training log so you can keep track of where you are in your training plan.

EXAMPLE:

BLOCK	CYCLE	WEEK 1	WEEK 2	WEEK 3	WEEK 4
A	1			OFF WORK	RACE 5k
	2	3 day Business Trip			
	3			Dental Procedure	
	4	4 day Weekend			RACE 10k

How to Use the CYCLE Training Plan Tool

The CYCLE planning tool is a place to plan your training in detail week by week.

1. From the BLOCK plan write the BLOCK letter.
2. Write the CYCLE number(s) from the BLOCK plan.
3. List all of the weeks in that CYCLE.
4. List all of the major events from the BLOCK planning tool.
5. Continue this process until you have listed all of the CYCLEs, and all of the weeks, and events in that BLOCK.
6. Create your daily training plan for each week in the CYCLE leading up to your event(s). Be sure to include OFF days or plan active rest.

EXAMPLE:

BLOCK __A__

CYCLE	WEEK	MON	TUE	WED	THUR	FRI	SAT	SUN
1	1	RUN	CF	OFF	RUN	CF	OFF	RUN
	2	CF	RUN	OFF	CF	RUN	OFF	RUN
OFF WORK	3	RUN	CF	OFF	RUN	CF	OFF	RUN
TAPER	4	CF	RUN	OFF	OFF	RUN	Race 5k	CF

How to Use the WEEKLY LOG

1. Write the BLOCK, CYCLE, and WEEK from the CYCLE planning tool. This will keep you on track with where you are in your training plan.

2. Write the date in the **DATE** box.

3. In the area below the day and date, write the workout(s) that you do for that day. Make sure to include all information about the workout; exercises, sets, reps, load, rounds, scaling, time....any information that will allow you to repeat the same workout at a later time. Also, write any notes regarding how the workout felt, problems with movements (the queues your trainer keeps yelling at you), PR's, actions that you take for recovery, etc.

4. At the end of the day, fill in the data for your **Recovery Factor.**

5. In the **NOTES** box, write any data or notes that do not apply to a given day. You can also calculate an average **Recovery Factor** metric to track your general recovery from week to week.

EXAMPLE:

BLOCK ___A___ CYCLE ___1___ WEEK ___2___

MONDAY   DATE 12/12/12

foam roller, dynamic stretching	Hydration (0-3) + 2 Roll(+1)
Back Squat 5x5	Nutrition (0-3) + 2 Mwod(+1)
5 rounds of:	Sleep (hrs) + 6 Stretch(+1)
200m row	Stress (0-3) 1 Yoga(+1)
7 DB Push Press @ #15	Tired(0-3) 2 Nap(+1)
21 KB Swings @ 16kg	Sore (0-3) 2 Msg(+1)
7 Knees to Chest	Sick (0-3) 0 Rest(+1)
	Injured (0-3) 0 Ice(+1)
18:27 - tired and sore!	Recovery Factor 8 Bwork(+1)

What is Recovery Factor?

The Recovery Factor is a number that gives you a general indication of how well you are recovering from your workouts. This number is composed of actions that, either bring you closer to recovery and ready to train (+), or further away from your goals (-). Proper hydration, good nutrition, adequate sleep, plus a number of **Recovery Actions**, go along way to helping you recover. Stress, fatigue, soreness, sickness, and injury will inhibit recovery.

The values are basically 0 to 3, with the exception of sleep where you would write the number of hours you slept. For positive factors, the higher the value the better. For negative factors, the opposite is true. Clearly, a Recovery Factor of 0 is bad.

The values are arbitrary, and will vary from person to person. When you chose a number, (positive or negative) be honest with yourself. Don't try to skew the Recovery Factor.

To find your Recovery Factor for a given day, simply total the positive factors (marked +), then subtract the negative factors (marked -).
In the example from the weekly log, the total for the positive factors is 13, including **Recovery Actions**. The total negative factors are 5.
13 - 5 = 8. 8 is the Recovery Factor for that day.

Continue to calculate your Recovery Factor throughout the week and trends will start to appear.

What are Recovery Actions?

Roll - Foam/PVC roller, ball of any type or size, Stick, doe roller, basically any soft tissue manipulation device.

Mwod - Kelly Starrett's Mobility WOD.

Stretch - Any stretching is good. Dynamic stretching is preferable. Jump Stretch band work is great.

Yoga - Any yoga or mobility class.

Nap - Take a nap. It doesn't matter how long.

Msg - Massage.

Rest - A rest day, can include active rest like walking or playing with your kids.

Ice - Using ice to reduce inflammation. Ice pack or ice bath, your choice.

Bwork - Body work. Any sort of body work from A.R.T. and Chiropractic, to Reiki and Rolfing, whatever helps you recover.

How to Use the
MAX EFFORT Template

Highly influenced by the excellent series of Max Effort Black Box articles by Coach Michael Rutherford (crossfitkc.com), this template can be used to track your strength gains using linear progression protocols.

The template is provided as an open format for you to write any combination of sets and reps whether they be 5 x 5, 3 x 8 or 6 x 2.

If you calculate your loads by percentage, the left column can be used to log these percentages.

If you should happen to not complete the number of reps required for a set, make sure you make a note of how many reps you actually completed next to the load for that set.

Example: *5 x 5 and 6 x 2 Back Squat*
EXAMPLE: Loads calculated for a 115 Kilo 1 RM

Set/%	DATE	DATE	DATE	DATE	DATE	DATE	DATE	DATE
5x5	2/22	2/30						
55%	63	63						
63%	72	72						
70%	81	81						
77%	89	89						
85%	98 (3)	98 (5)						
6x2	3/25	4/2						
	95	95						
	98	98						
	100	100						
	105	105						
	110	110						
	113 (1)	113 (2)						

How to Use the
BENCHMARK WORKOUT Log

In the Benchmark Workout Log section you can keep track of workouts and training events that you repeat frequently (ie. 2000m row), or any workout with a name (ie. Helen).

Make sure to record how you scaled the workout and any notes about the workout. You could also include the BLOCK, CYCLE, and week that you completed the workout.

EXAMPLE:

NAME	RX	Load/Scale	Time/Round
Helen			11/15/12
3 rounds of:			
400m run	24kg		12:53
21 kb swings		16 kg black band	PR!
12 pullups			B2C3W1

How to Use the
PERSONAL RECORD TRACKING

The Personal Record Tracking section is meant to celebrate all of your personal best efforts all in one place. Included on the page are some basic lifts to get you started. You can then enter any events or workouts that you want to track.

1. Enter the event, lift, or workout you want to track.
2. When you obtain a PR, enter the date. Then enter the tracking metric; load, time, distance, etc.

EXAMPLE:

	2/22/13	4/30/13	6/1/13			
Deadlift	98kg	105kg	115kg			

	1/25/13	3/11/13	5/10/13			
Back Squat	90kg	96kg	100kg			

	2/22/13	4/30/13	6/1/13			
Press	52kg	54kg	55kg			

The Training Log was created to help you plan, track, and document your progress on the journey to being the best athlete you can be.

If this Training Log was helpful to you, I would be so grateful for a 5 star review. It really helps.

If you have any suggestions on how I can improve this Log, please let me know at *humanstrengthcoach@gmail.com*.
I'd love to hear from you!

Find me on:

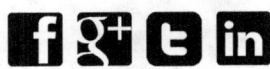

BLOCK ANNUAL TRAINING PLAN TOOL

BLOCK	CYCLE	WEEK 1	WEEK 2
		DATE	DATE
		DATE	DATE
		DATE	DATE
		DATE	DATE
		DATE	DATE
		DATE	DATE
		DATE	DATE
		DATE	DATE
		DATE	DATE
		DATE	DATE
		DATE	DATE
		DATE	DATE
		DATE	DATE
		DATE	DATE
		DATE	DATE
		DATE	DATE

BLOCK ANNUAL TRAINING PLAN TOOL

WEEK 3	WEEK 4	NOTES
DATE	DATE	
DATE	DATE	
DATE	DATE	
DATE	DATE	
DATE	DATE	
DATE	DATE	
DATE	DATE	
DATE	DATE	
DATE	DATE	
DATE	DATE	
DATE	DATE	
DATE	DATE	
DATE	DATE	
DATE	DATE	
DATE	DATE	
DATE	DATE	
DATE	DATE	
DATE	DATE	

BLOCK ANNUAL TRAINING PLAN TOOL

BLOCK	CYCLE	WEEK 1	WEEK 2
		DATE	DATE
		DATE	DATE
		DATE	DATE
		DATE	DATE
		DATE	DATE
		DATE	DATE
		DATE	DATE
		DATE	DATE
		DATE	DATE
		DATE	DATE
		DATE	DATE
		DATE	DATE
		DATE	DATE
		DATE	DATE
		DATE	DATE
		DATE	DATE
		DATE	DATE
		DATE	DATE

BLOCK ANNUAL TRAINING PLAN TOOL

WEEK 3   WEEK 4

DATE	DATE
DATE	DATE
DATE	DATE
DATE	DATE
DATE	DATE
DATE	DATE
DATE	DATE
DATE	DATE
DATE	DATE
DATE	DATE
DATE	DATE
DATE	DATE
DATE	DATE
DATE	DATE
DATE	DATE
DATE	DATE
DATE	DATE
DATE	DATE

BLOCK ANNUAL TRAINING PLAN TOOL

BLOCK	CYCLE	WEEK 1	WEEK 2
		DATE	DATE
		DATE	DATE
		DATE	DATE
		DATE	DATE
		DATE	DATE
		DATE	DATE
		DATE	DATE
		DATE	DATE
		DATE	DATE
		DATE	DATE
		DATE	DATE
		DATE	DATE
		DATE	DATE
		DATE	DATE
		DATE	DATE
		DATE	DATE

BLOCK ANNUAL TRAINING PLAN TOOL

WEEK 3	WEEK 4	NOTES
DATE	DATE	
DATE	DATE	
DATE	DATE	
DATE	DATE	
DATE	DATE	
DATE	DATE	
DATE	DATE	
DATE	DATE	
DATE	DATE	
DATE	DATE	
DATE	DATE	
DATE	DATE	
DATE	DATE	
DATE	DATE	
DATE	DATE	
DATE	DATE	

BLOCK _____

CYCLE	WEEK	MONDAY	TUESDAY	WEDNESDAY
		DATE	DATE	DATE
		DATE	DATE	DATE
		DATE	DATE	DATE
		DATE	DATE	DATE
		DATE	DATE	DATE
		DATE	DATE	DATE
		DATE	DATE	DATE
		DATE	DATE	DATE
		DATE	DATE	DATE
		DATE	DATE	DATE
		DATE	DATE	DATE
		DATE	DATE	DATE
		DATE	DATE	DATE
		DATE	DATE	DATE
		DATE	DATE	DATE
		DATE	DATE	DATE
		DATE	DATE	DATE
		DATE	DATE	DATE

CYCLE TRAINING PLAN TOOL

THURSDAY	FRIDAY	SATURDAY	SUNDAY
DATE	DATE	DATE	DATE
DATE	DATE	DATE	DATE
DATE	DATE	DATE	DATE
DATE	DATE	DATE	DATE
DATE	DATE	DATE	DATE
DATE	DATE	DATE	DATE
DATE	DATE	DATE	DATE
DATE	DATE	DATE	DATE
DATE	DATE	DATE	DATE
DATE	DATE	DATE	DATE
DATE	DATE	DATE	DATE
DATE	DATE	DATE	DATE
DATE	DATE	DATE	DATE
DATE	DATE	DATE	DATE
DATE	DATE	DATE	DATE
DATE	DATE	DATE	DATE
DATE	DATE	DATE	DATE

BLOCK _____

CYCLE	WEEK	MONDAY	TUESDAY	WEDNESDAY
		DATE	DATE	DATE
		DATE	DATE	DATE
		DATE	DATE	DATE
		DATE	DATE	DATE
		DATE	DATE	DATE
		DATE	DATE	DATE
		DATE	DATE	DATE
		DATE	DATE	DATE
		DATE	DATE	DATE
		DATE	DATE	DATE
		DATE	DATE	DATE
		DATE	DATE	DATE
		DATE	DATE	DATE
		DATE	DATE	DATE
		DATE	DATE	DATE
		DATE	DATE	DATE

CYCLE TRAINING PLAN TOOL

THURSDAY	FRIDAY	SATURDAY	SUNDAY
DATE	DATE	DATE	DATE
DATE	DATE	DATE	DATE
DATE	DATE	DATE	DATE
DATE	DATE	DATE	DATE
DATE	DATE	DATE	DATE
DATE	DATE	DATE	DATE
DATE	DATE	DATE	DATE
DATE	DATE	DATE	DATE
DATE	DATE	DATE	DATE
DATE	DATE	DATE	DATE
DATE	DATE	DATE	DATE
DATE	DATE	DATE	DATE
DATE	DATE	DATE	DATE
DATE	DATE	DATE	DATE
DATE	DATE	DATE	DATE
DATE	DATE	DATE	DATE

BLOCK _____

CYCLE	WEEK	MONDAY	TUESDAY	WEDNESDAY
		DATE	DATE	DATE
		DATE	DATE	DATE
		DATE	DATE	DATE
		DATE	DATE	DATE
		DATE	DATE	DATE
		DATE	DATE	DATE
		DATE	DATE	DATE
		DATE	DATE	DATE
		DATE	DATE	DATE
		DATE	DATE	DATE
		DATE	DATE	DATE
		DATE	DATE	DATE
		DATE	DATE	DATE
		DATE	DATE	DATE
		DATE	DATE	DATE
		DATE	DATE	DATE
		DATE	DATE	DATE
		DATE	DATE	DATE

CYCLE TRAINING PLAN TOOL

THURSDAY	FRIDAY	SATURDAY	SUNDAY
DATE	DATE	DATE	DATE
DATE	DATE	DATE	DATE
DATE	DATE	DATE	DATE
DATE	DATE	DATE	DATE
DATE	DATE	DATE	DATE
DATE	DATE	DATE	DATE
DATE	DATE	DATE	DATE
DATE	DATE	DATE	DATE
DATE	DATE	DATE	DATE
DATE	DATE	DATE	DATE
DATE	DATE	DATE	DATE
DATE	DATE	DATE	DATE
DATE	DATE	DATE	DATE
DATE	DATE	DATE	DATE
DATE	DATE	DATE	DATE
DATE	DATE	DATE	DATE

BLOCK _____

CYCLE	WEEK	MONDAY	TUESDAY	WEDNESDAY
		DATE	DATE	DATE
		DATE	DATE	DATE
		DATE	DATE	DATE
		DATE	DATE	DATE
		DATE	DATE	DATE
		DATE	DATE	DATE
		DATE	DATE	DATE
		DATE	DATE	DATE
		DATE	DATE	DATE
		DATE	DATE	DATE
		DATE	DATE	DATE
		DATE	DATE	DATE
		DATE	DATE	DATE
		DATE	DATE	DATE
		DATE	DATE	DATE
		DATE	DATE	DATE
		DATE	DATE	DATE
		DATE	DATE	DATE

CYCLE TRAINING PLAN TOOL

THURSDAY	FRIDAY	SATURDAY	SUNDAY
DATE	DATE	DATE	DATE
DATE	DATE	DATE	DATE
DATE	DATE	DATE	DATE
DATE	DATE	DATE	DATE
DATE	DATE	DATE	DATE
DATE	DATE	DATE	DATE
DATE	DATE	DATE	DATE
DATE	DATE	DATE	DATE
DATE	DATE	DATE	DATE
DATE	DATE	DATE	DATE
DATE	DATE	DATE	DATE
DATE	DATE	DATE	DATE
DATE	DATE	DATE	DATE
DATE	DATE	DATE	DATE
DATE	DATE	DATE	DATE
DATE	DATE	DATE	DATE
DATE	DATE	DATE	DATE

BLOCK _____

CYCLE	WEEK	MONDAY	TUESDAY	WEDNESDAY
		DATE	DATE	DATE
		DATE	DATE	DATE
		DATE	DATE	DATE
		DATE	DATE	DATE
		DATE	DATE	DATE
		DATE	DATE	DATE
		DATE	DATE	DATE
		DATE	DATE	DATE
		DATE	DATE	DATE
		DATE	DATE	DATE
		DATE	DATE	DATE
		DATE	DATE	DATE
		DATE	DATE	DATE
		DATE	DATE	DATE
		DATE	DATE	DATE
		DATE	DATE	DATE
		DATE	DATE	DATE

CYCLE TRAINING PLAN TOOL

THURSDAY	FRIDAY	SATURDAY	SUNDAY
DATE	DATE	DATE	DATE
DATE	DATE	DATE	DATE
DATE	DATE	DATE	DATE
DATE	DATE	DATE	DATE
DATE	DATE	DATE	DATE
DATE	DATE	DATE	DATE
DATE	DATE	DATE	DATE
DATE	DATE	DATE	DATE
DATE	DATE	DATE	DATE
DATE	DATE	DATE	DATE
DATE	DATE	DATE	DATE
DATE	DATE	DATE	DATE
DATE	DATE	DATE	DATE
DATE	DATE	DATE	DATE
DATE	DATE	DATE	DATE
DATE	DATE	DATE	DATE
DATE	DATE	DATE	DATE

BLOCK _____

CYCLE	WEEK	MONDAY	TUESDAY	WEDNESDAY
		DATE	DATE	DATE
		DATE	DATE	DATE
		DATE	DATE	DATE
		DATE	DATE	DATE
		DATE	DATE	DATE
		DATE	DATE	DATE
		DATE	DATE	DATE
		DATE	DATE	DATE
		DATE	DATE	DATE
		DATE	DATE	DATE
		DATE	DATE	DATE
		DATE	DATE	DATE
		DATE	DATE	DATE
		DATE	DATE	DATE
		DATE	DATE	DATE
		DATE	DATE	DATE
		DATE	DATE	DATE

CYCLE TRAINING PLAN TOOL

THURSDAY	FRIDAY	SATURDAY	SUNDAY
DATE	DATE	DATE	DATE
DATE	DATE	DATE	DATE
DATE	DATE	DATE	DATE
DATE	DATE	DATE	DATE
DATE	DATE	DATE	DATE
DATE	DATE	DATE	DATE
DATE	DATE	DATE	DATE
DATE	DATE	DATE	DATE
DATE	DATE	DATE	DATE
DATE	DATE	DATE	DATE
DATE	DATE	DATE	DATE
DATE	DATE	DATE	DATE
DATE	DATE	DATE	DATE
DATE	DATE	DATE	DATE
DATE	DATE	DATE	DATE
DATE	DATE	DATE	DATE
DATE	DATE	DATE	DATE
DATE	DATE	DATE	DATE

BLOCK _____ CYCLE _____ WEEK _____

MONDAY   DATE

Hydration (0-3) + _____	Roll(+1)
Nutrition (0-3) + _____	Mwod(+1)
Sleep (hrs) + _____	Stretch(+1)
Stress (0-3)	Yoga(+1)
Tired(0-3)	Nap(+1)
Sore (0-3)	Msg(+1)
Sick (0-3)	Rest(+1)
Injured (0-3)	Ice(+1)
Recovery Factor	Bwork(+1)

TUESDAY   DATE

Hydration (0-3) + _____	Roll(+1)
Nutrition (0-3) + _____	Mwod(+1)
Sleep (hrs) + _____	Stretch(+1)
Stress (0-3)	Yoga(+1)
Tired(0-3)	Nap(+1)
Sore (0-3)	Msg(+1)
Sick (0-3)	Rest(+1)
Injured (0-3)	Ice(+1)
Recovery Factor	Bwork(+1)

WEDNESDAY   DATE

Hydration (0-3) + _____	Roll(+1)
Nutrition (0-3) + _____	Mwod(+1)
Sleep (hrs) + _____	Stretch(+1)
Stress (0-3)	Yoga(+1)
Tired(0-3)	Nap(+1)
Sore (0-3)	Msg(+1)
Sick (0-3)	Rest(+1)
Injured (0-3)	Ice(+1)
Recovery Factor	Bwork(+1)

THURSDAY   DATE

Hydration (0-3) + _____	Roll(+1)
Nutrition (0-3) + _____	Mwod(+1)
Sleep (hrs) + _____	Stretch(+1)
Stress (0-3)	Yoga(+1)
Tired(0-3)	Nap(+1)
Sore (0-3)	Msg(+1)
Sick (0-3)	Rest(+1)
Injured (0-3)	Ice(+1)
Recovery Factor	Bwork(+1)

WEEKLY LOG

FRIDAY   DATE _____

_____

_____

_____

_____

_____

_____

_____

_____

_____

Hydration (0-3) + _____	Roll(+1)
Nutrition (0-3) + _____	Mwod(+1)
Sleep (hrs) + _____	Stretch(+1)
Stress (0-3)	Yoga(+1)
Tired(0-3)	Nap(+1)
Sore (0-3)	Msg(+1)
Sick (0-3)	Rest(+1)
Injured (0-3)	Ice(+1)
Recovery Factor	Bwork(+1)

SATURDAY   DATE _____

_____

_____

_____

_____

_____

_____

_____

_____

Hydration (0-3) + _____	Roll(+1)
Nutrition (0-3) + _____	Mwod(+1)
Sleep (hrs) + _____	Stretch(+1)
Stress (0-3)	Yoga(+1)
Tired(0-3)	Nap(+1)
Sore (0-3)	Msg(+1)
Sick (0-3)	Rest(+1)
Injured (0-3)	Ice(+1)
Recovery Factor	Bwork(+1)

SUNDAY   DATE _____

_____

_____

_____

_____

_____

_____

_____

_____

Hydration (0-3) + _____	Roll(+1)
Nutrition (0-3) + _____	Mwod(+1)
Sleep (hrs) + _____	Stretch(+1)
Stress (0-3)	Yoga(+1)
Tired(0-3)	Nap(+1)
Sore (0-3)	Msg(+1)
Sick (0-3)	Rest(+1)
Injured (0-3)	Ice(+1)
Recovery Factor	Bwork(+1)

NOTES

Weekly RF Tracking

M _____

T _____

W _____

T _____

F _____

S _____

S _____

Average
Recovery Factor _____

BLOCK _____ CYCLE _____ WEEK _____

MONDAY   DATE

_____
_____ Hydration (0-3) +_____ Roll(+1)
_____ Nutrition (0-3) +_____ Mwod(+1)
_____ Sleep (hrs)   +_____ Stretch(+1)
_____ Stress (0-3)   Yoga(+1)
_____ Tired(0-3)   Nap(+1)
_____ Sore (0-3)   Msg(+1)
_____ Sick (0-3)   Rest(+1)
_____ Injured (0-3)   Ice(+1)
                               Recovery Factor   Bwork(+1)

TUESDAY   DATE

_____
_____ Hydration (0-3) +_____ Roll(+1)
_____ Nutrition (0-3) +_____ Mwod(+1)
_____ Sleep (hrs)   +_____ Stretch(+1)
_____ Stress (0-3)   Yoga(+1)
_____ Tired(0-3)   Nap(+1)
_____ Sore (0-3)   Msg(+1)
_____ Sick (0-3)   Rest(+1)
_____ Injured (0-3)   Ice(+1)
                               Recovery Factor   Bwork(+1)

WEDNESDAY   DATE

_____
_____ Hydration (0-3) +_____ Roll(+1)
_____ Nutrition (0-3) +_____ Mwod(+1)
_____ Sleep (hrs)   +_____ Stretch(+1)
_____ Stress (0-3)   Yoga(+1)
_____ Tired(0-3)   Nap(+1)
_____ Sore (0-3)   Msg(+1)
_____ Sick (0-3)   Rest(+1)
_____ Injured (0-3)   Ice(+1)
                               Recovery Factor   Bwork(+1)

THURSDAY   DATE

_____
_____ Hydration (0-3) +_____ Roll(+1)
_____ Nutrition (0-3) +_____ Mwod(+1)
_____ Sleep (hrs)   +_____ Stretch(+1)
_____ Stress (0-3)   Yoga(+1)
_____ Tired(0-3)   Nap(+1)
_____ Sore (0-3)   Msg(+1)
_____ Sick (0-3)   Rest(+1)
_____ Injured (0-3)   Ice(+1)
                               Recovery Factor   Bwork(+1)

WEEKLY LOG

FRIDAY   DATE

_____

Hydration (0-3) + _____		Roll(+1)
Nutrition (0-3) + _____		Mwod(+1)
Sleep (hrs) + _____		Stretch(+1)
Stress (0-3)		Yoga(+1)
Tired(0-3)		Nap(+1)
Sore (0-3)		Msg(+1)
Sick (0-3)		Rest(+1)
Injured (0-3)		Ice(+1)
Recovery Factor		Bwork(+1)

SATURDAY   DATE

_____

Hydration (0-3) + _____		Roll(+1)
Nutrition (0-3) + _____		Mwod(+1)
Sleep (hrs) + _____		Stretch(+1)
Stress (0-3)		Yoga(+1)
Tired(0-3)		Nap(+1)
Sore (0-3)		Msg(+1)
Sick (0-3)		Rest(+1)
Injured (0-3)		Ice(+1)
Recovery Factor		Bwork(+1)

SUNDAY   DATE

_____

Hydration (0-3) + _____		Roll(+1)
Nutrition (0-3) + _____		Mwod(+1)
Sleep (hrs) + _____		Stretch(+1)
Stress (0-3)		Yoga(+1)
Tired(0-3)		Nap(+1)
Sore (0-3)		Msg(+1)
Sick (0-3)		Rest(+1)
Injured (0-3)		Ice(+1)
Recovery Factor		Bwork(+1)

NOTES

Weekly RF Tracking

M _____
T _____
W _____
T _____
F _____
S _____
S _____
Average
Recovery Factor _____

BLOCK _____ CYCLE _____ WEEK _____

MONDAY   DATE _____

_____
_____
_____
_____
_____
_____
_____
_____

Hydration (0-3) +_____ Roll(+1)
Nutrition (0-3) +_____ Mwod(+1)
Sleep (hrs)   +_____ Stretch(+1)
Stress (0-3)   Yoga(+1)
Tired(0-3)   Nap(+1)
Sore (0-3)   Msg(+1)
Sick (0-3)   Rest(+1)
Injured (0-3)   Ice(+1)
Recovery Factor   Bwork(+1)

TUESDAY   DATE _____

_____
_____
_____
_____
_____
_____
_____
_____

Hydration (0-3) +_____ Roll(+1)
Nutrition (0-3) +_____ Mwod(+1)
Sleep (hrs)   +_____ Stretch(+1)
Stress (0-3)   Yoga(+1)
Tired(0-3)   Nap(+1)
Sore (0-3)   Msg(+1)
Sick (0-3)   Rest(+1)
Injured (0-3)   Ice(+1)
Recovery Factor   Bwork(+1)

WEDNESDAY   DATE _____

_____
_____
_____
_____
_____
_____
_____
_____

Hydration (0-3) +_____ Roll(+1)
Nutrition (0-3) +_____ Mwod(+1)
Sleep (hrs)   +_____ Stretch(+1)
Stress (0-3)   Yoga(+1)
Tired(0-3)   Nap(+1)
Sore (0-3)   Msg(+1)
Sick (0-3)   Rest(+1)
Injured (0-3)   Ice(+1)
Recovery Factor   Bwork(+1)

THURSDAY   DATE _____

_____
_____
_____
_____
_____
_____
_____
_____

Hydration (0-3) +_____ Roll(+1)
Nutrition (0-3) +_____ Mwod(+1)
Sleep (hrs)   +_____ Stretch(+1)
Stress (0-3)   Yoga(+1)
Tired(0-3)   Nap(+1)
Sore (0-3)   Msg(+1)
Sick (0-3)   Rest(+1)
Injured (0-3)   Ice(+1)
Recovery Factor   Bwork(+1)

WEEKLY LOG

FRIDAY   DATE _____

_____

Hydration (0-3) +_____	Roll(+1)
Nutrition (0-3) +_____	Mwod(+1)
Sleep (hrs) +_____	Stretch(+1)
Stress (0-3)	Yoga(+1)
Tired(0-3)	Nap(+1)
Sore (0-3)	Msg(+1)
Sick (0-3)	Rest(+1)
Injured (0-3)	Ice(+1)
Recovery Factor	Bwork(+1)

SATURDAY   DATE _____

_____

Hydration (0-3) +_____	Roll(+1)
Nutrition (0-3) +_____	Mwod(+1)
Sleep (hrs) +_____	Stretch(+1)
Stress (0-3)	Yoga(+1)
Tired(0-3)	Nap(+1)
Sore (0-3)	Msg(+1)
Sick (0-3)	Rest(+1)
Injured (0-3)	Ice(+1)
Recovery Factor	Bwork(+1)

SUNDAY   DATE _____

_____

Hydration (0-3) +_____	Roll(+1)
Nutrition (0-3) +_____	Mwod(+1)
Sleep (hrs) +_____	Stretch(+1)
Stress (0-3)	Yoga(+1)
Tired(0-3)	Nap(+1)
Sore (0-3)	Msg(+1)
Sick (0-3)	Rest(+1)
Injured (0-3)	Ice(+1)
Recovery Factor	Bwork(+1)

NOTES

Weekly RF Tracking

M _____
T _____
W _____
T _____
F _____
S _____
S _____
Average
Recovery Factor _____

BLOCK _____ CYCLE _____ WEEK _____

MONDAY   DATE

_____

Hydration (0-3) + _____		Roll(+1)
Nutrition (0-3) + _____		Mwod(+1)
Sleep (hrs) + _____		Stretch(+1)
Stress (0-3)		Yoga(+1)
Tired(0-3)		Nap(+1)
Sore (0-3)		Msg(+1)
Sick (0-3)		Rest(+1)
Injured (0-3)		Ice(+1)
Recovery Factor		Bwork(+1)

TUESDAY   DATE

_____

Hydration (0-3) + _____		Roll(+1)
Nutrition (0-3) + _____		Mwod(+1)
Sleep (hrs) + _____		Stretch(+1)
Stress (0-3)		Yoga(+1)
Tired(0-3)		Nap(+1)
Sore (0-3)		Msg(+1)
Sick (0-3)		Rest(+1)
Injured (0-3)		Ice(+1)
Recovery Factor		Bwork(+1)

WEDNESDAY   DATE

_____

Hydration (0-3) + _____		Roll(+1)
Nutrition (0-3) + _____		Mwod(+1)
Sleep (hrs) + _____		Stretch(+1)
Stress (0-3)		Yoga(+1)
Tired(0-3)		Nap(+1)
Sore (0-3)		Msg(+1)
Sick (0-3)		Rest(+1)
Injured (0-3)		Ice(+1)
Recovery Factor		Bwork(+1)

THURSDAY   DATE

_____

Hydration (0-3) + _____		Roll(+1)
Nutrition (0-3) + _____		Mwod(+1)
Sleep (hrs) + _____		Stretch(+1)
Stress (0-3)		Yoga(+1)
Tired(0-3)		Nap(+1)
Sore (0-3)		Msg(+1)
Sick (0-3)		Rest(+1)
Injured (0-3)		Ice(+1)
Recovery Factor		Bwork(+1)

WEEKLY LOG

FRIDAY   DATE

_____

Hydration (0-3) + _____	Roll(+1)
Nutrition (0-3) + _____	Mwod(+1)
Sleep (hrs) + _____	Stretch(+1)
Stress (0-3)	Yoga(+1)
Tired(0-3)	Nap(+1)
Sore (0-3)	Msg(+1)
Sick (0-3)	Rest(+1)
Injured (0-3)	Ice(+1)
Recovery Factor	Bwork(+1)

SATURDAY   DATE

_____

Hydration (0-3) + _____	Roll(+1)
Nutrition (0-3) + _____	Mwod(+1)
Sleep (hrs) + _____	Stretch(+1)
Stress (0-3)	Yoga(+1)
Tired(0-3)	Nap(+1)
Sore (0-3)	Msg(+1)
Sick (0-3)	Rest(+1)
Injured (0-3)	Ice(+1)
Recovery Factor	Bwork(+1)

SUNDAY   DATE

_____

Hydration (0-3) + _____	Roll(+1)
Nutrition (0-3) + _____	Mwod(+1)
Sleep (hrs) + _____	Stretch(+1)
Stress (0-3)	Yoga(+1)
Tired(0-3)	Nap(+1)
Sore (0-3)	Msg(+1)
Sick (0-3)	Rest(+1)
Injured (0-3)	Ice(+1)
Recovery Factor	Bwork(+1)

NOTES

Weekly RF Tracking

M _____
T _____
W _____
T _____
F _____
S _____
S _____
Average
Recovery Factor _____

BLOCK _____ CYCLE _____ WEEK _____

MONDAY   DATE

_____

Hydration (0-3) +_____	Roll(+1)
Nutrition (0-3) +_____	Mwod(+1)
Sleep (hrs) +_____	Stretch(+1)
Stress (0-3)	Yoga(+1)
Tired(0-3)	Nap(+1)
Sore (0-3)	Msg(+1)
Sick (0-3)	Rest(+1)
Injured (0-3)	Ice(+1)
Recovery Factor	Bwork(+1)

TUESDAY   DATE

_____

Hydration (0-3) +_____	Roll(+1)
Nutrition (0-3) +_____	Mwod(+1)
Sleep (hrs) +_____	Stretch(+1)
Stress (0-3)	Yoga(+1)
Tired(0-3)	Nap(+1)
Sore (0-3)	Msg(+1)
Sick (0-3)	Rest(+1)
Injured (0-3)	Ice(+1)
Recovery Factor	Bwork(+1)

WEDNESDAY   DATE

_____

Hydration (0-3) +_____	Roll(+1)
Nutrition (0-3) +_____	Mwod(+1)
Sleep (hrs) +_____	Stretch(+1)
Stress (0-3)	Yoga(+1)
Tired(0-3)	Nap(+1)
Sore (0-3)	Msg(+1)
Sick (0-3)	Rest(+1)
Injured (0-3)	Ice(+1)
Recovery Factor	Bwork(+1)

THURSDAY   DATE

_____

Hydration (0-3) +_____	Roll(+1)
Nutrition (0-3) +_____	Mwod(+1)
Sleep (hrs) +_____	Stretch(+1)
Stress (0-3)	Yoga(+1)
Tired(0-3)	Nap(+1)
Sore (0-3)	Msg(+1)
Sick (0-3)	Rest(+1)
Injured (0-3)	Ice(+1)
Recovery Factor	Bwork(+1)

WEEKLY LOG

FRIDAY   DATE

_____

Hydration (0-3) +_____ Roll(+1)
Nutrition (0-3) +_____ Mwod(+1)
Sleep (hrs) +_____ Stretch(+1)
Stress (0-3)   Yoga(+1)
Tired(0-3)   Nap(+1)
Sore (0-3)   Msg(+1)
Sick (0-3)   Rest(+1)
Injured (0-3)   Ice(+1)
Recovery Factor   Bwork(+1)

SATURDAY   DATE

_____

Hydration (0-3) +_____ Roll(+1)
Nutrition (0-3) +_____ Mwod(+1)
Sleep (hrs) +_____ Stretch(+1)
Stress (0-3)   Yoga(+1)
Tired(0-3)   Nap(+1)
Sore (0-3)   Msg(+1)
Sick (0-3)   Rest(+1)
Injured (0-3)   Ice(+1)
Recovery Factor   Bwork(+1)

SUNDAY   DATE

_____

Hydration (0-3) +_____ Roll(+1)
Nutrition (0-3) +_____ Mwod(+1)
Sleep (hrs) +_____ Stretch(+1)
Stress (0-3)   Yoga(+1)
Tired(0-3)   Nap(+1)
Sore (0-3)   Msg(+1)
Sick (0-3)   Rest(+1)
Injured (0-3)   Ice(+1)
Recovery Factor   Bwork(+1)

NOTES

Weekly RF Tracking
M _____
T _____
W _____
T _____
F _____
S _____
S _____
Average
Recovery Factor _____

BLOCK _____ CYCLE _____ WEEK _____

MONDAY   DATE

Hydration (0-3) + _____	Roll(+1)
Nutrition (0-3) + _____	Mwod(+1)
Sleep (hrs) + _____	Stretch(+1)
Stress (0-3)	Yoga(+1)
Tired(0-3)	Nap(+1)
Sore (0-3)	Msg(+1)
Sick (0-3)	Rest(+1)
Injured (0-3)	Ice(+1)
Recovery Factor	Bwork(+1)

TUESDAY   DATE

Hydration (0-3) + _____	Roll(+1)
Nutrition (0-3) + _____	Mwod(+1)
Sleep (hrs) + _____	Stretch(+1)
Stress (0-3)	Yoga(+1)
Tired(0-3)	Nap(+1)
Sore (0-3)	Msg(+1)
Sick (0-3)	Rest(+1)
Injured (0-3)	Ice(+1)
Recovery Factor	Bwork(+1)

WEDNESDAY   DATE

Hydration (0-3) + _____	Roll(+1)
Nutrition (0-3) + _____	Mwod(+1)
Sleep (hrs) + _____	Stretch(+1)
Stress (0-3)	Yoga(+1)
Tired(0-3)	Nap(+1)
Sore (0-3)	Msg(+1)
Sick (0-3)	Rest(+1)
Injured (0-3)	Ice(+1)
Recovery Factor	Bwork(+1)

THURSDAY   DATE

Hydration (0-3) + _____	Roll(+1)
Nutrition (0-3) + _____	Mwod(+1)
Sleep (hrs) + _____	Stretch(+1)
Stress (0-3)	Yoga(+1)
Tired(0-3)	Nap(+1)
Sore (0-3)	Msg(+1)
Sick (0-3)	Rest(+1)
Injured (0-3)	Ice(+1)
Recovery Factor	Bwork(+1)

WEEKLY LOG

FRIDAY   DATE

_____

_____

_____

_____

_____

_____

_____

_____

_____

Hydration (0-3) + _____		Roll(+1)
Nutrition (0-3) + _____		Mwod(+1)
Sleep (hrs) + _____		Stretch(+1)
Stress (0-3)		Yoga(+1)
Tired(0-3)		Nap(+1)
Sore (0-3)		Msg(+1)
Sick (0-3)		Rest(+1)
Injured (0-3)		Ice(+1)
Recovery Factor		Bwork(+1)

SATURDAY   DATE

_____

_____

_____

_____

_____

_____

_____

_____

_____

Hydration (0-3) + _____		Roll(+1)
Nutrition (0-3) + _____		Mwod(+1)
Sleep (hrs) + _____		Stretch(+1)
Stress (0-3)		Yoga(+1)
Tired(0-3)		Nap(+1)
Sore (0-3)		Msg(+1)
Sick (0-3)		Rest(+1)
Injured (0-3)		Ice(+1)
Recovery Factor		Bwork(+1)

SUNDAY   DATE

_____

_____

_____

_____

_____

_____

_____

_____

_____

Hydration (0-3) + _____		Roll(+1)
Nutrition (0-3) + _____		Mwod(+1)
Sleep (hrs) + _____		Stretch(+1)
Stress (0-3)		Yoga(+1)
Tired(0-3)		Nap(+1)
Sore (0-3)		Msg(+1)
Sick (0-3)		Rest(+1)
Injured (0-3)		Ice(+1)
Recovery Factor		Bwork(+1)

NOTES

Weekly RF Tracking

M _____

T _____

W _____

T _____

F _____

S _____

S _____

Average
Recovery Factor _____

BLOCK _____ CYCLE _____ WEEK _____

MONDAY _____ DATE _____

_____

Hydration (0-3) + _____	Roll(+1)
Nutrition (0-3) + _____	Mwod(+1)
Sleep (hrs) + _____	Stretch(+1)
Stress (0-3)	Yoga(+1)
Tired(0-3)	Nap(+1)
Sore (0-3)	Msg(+1)
Sick (0-3)	Rest(+1)
Injured (0-3)	Ice(+1)
Recovery Factor	Bwork(+1)

TUESDAY _____ DATE _____

_____

Hydration (0-3) + _____	Roll(+1)
Nutrition (0-3) + _____	Mwod(+1)
Sleep (hrs) + _____	Stretch(+1)
Stress (0-3)	Yoga(+1)
Tired(0-3)	Nap(+1)
Sore (0-3)	Msg(+1)
Sick (0-3)	Rest(+1)
Injured (0-3)	Ice(+1)
Recovery Factor	Bwork(+1)

WEDNESDAY _____ DATE _____

_____

Hydration (0-3) + _____	Roll(+1)
Nutrition (0-3) + _____	Mwod(+1)
Sleep (hrs) + _____	Stretch(+1)
Stress (0-3)	Yoga(+1)
Tired(0-3)	Nap(+1)
Sore (0-3)	Msg(+1)
Sick (0-3)	Rest(+1)
Injured (0-3)	Ice(+1)
Recovery Factor	Bwork(+1)

THURSDAY _____ DATE _____

_____

Hydration (0-3) + _____	Roll(+1)
Nutrition (0-3) + _____	Mwod(+1)
Sleep (hrs) + _____	Stretch(+1)
Stress (0-3)	Yoga(+1)
Tired(0-3)	Nap(+1)
Sore (0-3)	Msg(+1)
Sick (0-3)	Rest(+1)
Injured (0-3)	Ice(+1)
Recovery Factor	Bwork(+1)

WEEKLY LOG

FRIDAY   DATE _____

_____

_____

_____

_____

_____

_____

_____

_____

_____

Hydration (0-3) +_____   Roll(+1)

Nutrition (0-3) +_____   Mwod(+1)

Sleep (hrs)   +_____   Stretch(+1)

Stress (0-3)   Yoga(+1)

Tired(0-3)   Nap(+1)

Sore (0-3)   Msg(+1)

Sick (0-3)   Rest(+1)

Injured (0-3)   Ice(+1)

Recovery Factor   Bwork(+1)

SATURDAY   DATE _____

_____

_____

_____

_____

_____

_____

_____

_____

Hydration (0-3) +_____   Roll(+1)

Nutrition (0-3) +_____   Mwod(+1)

Sleep (hrs)   +_____   Stretch(+1)

Stress (0-3)   Yoga(+1)

Tired(0-3)   Nap(+1)

Sore (0-3)   Msg(+1)

Sick (0-3)   Rest(+1)

Injured (0-3)   Ice(+1)

Recovery Factor   Bwork(+1)

SUNDAY   DATE _____

_____

_____

_____

_____

_____

_____

_____

_____

_____

Hydration (0-3) +_____   Roll(+1)

Nutrition (0-3) +_____   Mwod(+1)

Sleep (hrs)   +_____   Stretch(+1)

Stress (0-3)   Yoga(+1)

Tired(0-3)   Nap(+1)

Sore (0-3)   Msg(+1)

Sick (0-3)   Rest(+1)

Injured (0-3)   Ice(+1)

Recovery Factor   Bwork(+1)

NOTES

Weekly RF Tracking

M _____

T _____

W _____

T _____

F _____

S _____

S _____

Average
Recovery Factor _____

BLOCK _____ CYCLE _____ WEEK _____

MONDAY   DATE _____

_____
_____
_____
_____
_____
_____
_____
_____
_____

Hydration (0-3) +_____		Roll(+1)
Nutrition (0-3) +_____		Mwod(+1)
Sleep (hrs) +_____		Stretch(+1)
Stress (0-3)		Yoga(+1)
Tired(0-3)		Nap(+1)
Sore (0-3)		Msg(+1)
Sick (0-3)		Rest(+1)
Injured (0-3)		Ice(+1)
Recovery Factor		Bwork(+1)

TUESDAY   DATE _____

_____
_____
_____
_____
_____
_____
_____
_____
_____

Hydration (0-3) +_____		Roll(+1)
Nutrition (0-3) +_____		Mwod(+1)
Sleep (hrs) +_____		Stretch(+1)
Stress (0-3)		Yoga(+1)
Tired(0-3)		Nap(+1)
Sore (0-3)		Msg(+1)
Sick (0-3)		Rest(+1)
Injured (0-3)		Ice(+1)
Recovery Factor		Bwork(+1)

WEDNESDAY   DATE _____

_____
_____
_____
_____
_____
_____
_____
_____
_____

Hydration (0-3) +_____		Roll(+1)
Nutrition (0-3) +_____		Mwod(+1)
Sleep (hrs) +_____		Stretch(+1)
Stress (0-3)		Yoga(+1)
Tired(0-3)		Nap(+1)
Sore (0-3)		Msg(+1)
Sick (0-3)		Rest(+1)
Injured (0-3)		Ice(+1)
Recovery Factor		Bwork(+1)

THURSDAY   DATE _____

_____
_____
_____
_____
_____
_____
_____
_____
_____

Hydration (0-3) +_____		Roll(+1)
Nutrition (0-3) +_____		Mwod(+1)
Sleep (hrs) +_____		Stretch(+1)
Stress (0-3)		Yoga(+1)
Tired(0-3)		Nap(+1)
Sore (0-3)		Msg(+1)
Sick (0-3)		Rest(+1)
Injured (0-3)		Ice(+1)
Recovery Factor		Bwork(+1)

WEEKLY LOG

FRIDAY   DATE _____

_____

_____

_____

_____

_____

_____

_____

_____

Hydration (0-3) +_____	Roll(+1)
Nutrition (0-3) +_____	Mwod(+1)
Sleep (hrs) +_____	Stretch(+1)
Stress (0-3)	Yoga(+1)
Tired(0-3)	Nap(+1)
Sore (0-3)	Msg(+1)
Sick (0-3)	Rest(+1)
Injured (0-3)	Ice(+1)
Recovery Factor	Bwork(+1)

SATURDAY   DATE _____

_____

_____

_____

_____

_____

_____

_____

_____

Hydration (0-3) +_____	Roll(+1)
Nutrition (0-3) +_____	Mwod(+1)
Sleep (hrs) +_____	Stretch(+1)
Stress (0-3)	Yoga(+1)
Tired(0-3)	Nap(+1)
Sore (0-3)	Msg(+1)
Sick (0-3)	Rest(+1)
Injured (0-3)	Ice(+1)
Recovery Factor	Bwork(+1)

SUNDAY   DATE _____

_____

_____

_____

_____

_____

_____

_____

_____

Hydration (0-3) +_____	Roll(+1)
Nutrition (0-3) +_____	Mwod(+1)
Sleep (hrs) +_____	Stretch(+1)
Stress (0-3)	Yoga(+1)
Tired(0-3)	Nap(+1)
Sore (0-3)	Msg(+1)
Sick (0-3)	Rest(+1)
Injured (0-3)	Ice(+1)
Recovery Factor	Bwork(+1)

NOTES

Weekly RF Tracking

M _____

T _____

W _____

T _____

F _____

S _____

S _____

Average
Recovery Factor _____

BLOCK _____ CYCLE _____ WEEK _____

MONDAY   DATE _____

_____

_____

_____

_____

_____

_____

_____

_____

Hydration (0-3) +_____	Roll(+1)
Nutrition (0-3) +_____	Mwod(+1)
Sleep (hrs) +_____	Stretch(+1)
Stress (0-3)	Yoga(+1)
Tired(0-3)	Nap(+1)
Sore (0-3)	Msg(+1)
Sick (0-3)	Rest(+1)
Injured (0-3)	Ice(+1)
Recovery Factor	Bwork(+1)

TUESDAY   DATE _____

_____

_____

_____

_____

_____

_____

_____

_____

Hydration (0-3) +_____	Roll(+1)
Nutrition (0-3) +_____	Mwod(+1)
Sleep (hrs) +_____	Stretch(+1)
Stress (0-3)	Yoga(+1)
Tired(0-3)	Nap(+1)
Sore (0-3)	Msg(+1)
Sick (0-3)	Rest(+1)
Injured (0-3)	Ice(+1)
Recovery Factor	Bwork(+1)

WEDNESDAY   DATE _____

_____

_____

_____

_____

_____

_____

_____

_____

Hydration (0-3) +_____	Roll(+1)
Nutrition (0-3) +_____	Mwod(+1)
Sleep (hrs) +_____	Stretch(+1)
Stress (0-3)	Yoga(+1)
Tired(0-3)	Nap(+1)
Sore (0-3)	Msg(+1)
Sick (0-3)	Rest(+1)
Injured (0-3)	Ice(+1)
Recovery Factor	Bwork(+1)

THURSDAY   DATE _____

_____

_____

_____

_____

_____

_____

_____

_____

Hydration (0-3) +_____	Roll(+1)
Nutrition (0-3) +_____	Mwod(+1)
Sleep (hrs) +_____	Stretch(+1)
Stress (0-3)	Yoga(+1)
Tired(0-3)	Nap(+1)
Sore (0-3)	Msg(+1)
Sick (0-3)	Rest(+1)
Injured (0-3)	Ice(+1)
Recovery Factor	Bwork(+1)

WEEKLY LOG

FRIDAY   DATE

_____

Hydration (0-3) +_____	Roll(+1)
Nutrition (0-3) +_____	Mwod(+1)
Sleep (hrs) +_____	Stretch(+1)
Stress (0-3)	Yoga(+1)
Tired(0-3)	Nap(+1)
Sore (0-3)	Msg(+1)
Sick (0-3)	Rest(+1)
Injured (0-3)	Ice(+1)
Recovery Factor	Bwork(+1)

SATURDAY   DATE

_____

Hydration (0-3) +_____	Roll(+1)
Nutrition (0-3) +_____	Mwod(+1)
Sleep (hrs) +_____	Stretch(+1)
Stress (0-3)	Yoga(+1)
Tired(0-3)	Nap(+1)
Sore (0-3)	Msg(+1)
Sick (0-3)	Rest(+1)
Injured (0-3)	Ice(+1)
Recovery Factor	Bwork(+1)

SUNDAY   DATE

_____

Hydration (0-3) +_____	Roll(+1)
Nutrition (0-3) +_____	Mwod(+1)
Sleep (hrs) +_____	Stretch(+1)
Stress (0-3)	Yoga(+1)
Tired(0-3)	Nap(+1)
Sore (0-3)	Msg(+1)
Sick (0-3)	Rest(+1)
Injured (0-3)	Ice(+1)
Recovery Factor	Bwork(+1)

NOTES

Weekly RF Tracking

M _____
T _____
W _____
T _____
F _____
S _____
S _____
Average
Recovery Factor _____

BLOCK _____ CYCLE _____ WEEK _____

MONDAY   DATE

	Hydration (0-3) +_____	Roll(+1)
	Nutrition (0-3) +_____	Mwod(+1)
	Sleep (hrs) +_____	Stretch(+1)
	Stress (0-3)	Yoga(+1)
	Tired(0-3)	Nap(+1)
	Sore (0-3)	Msg(+1)
	Sick (0-3)	Rest(+1)
	Injured (0-3)	Ice(+1)
	Recovery Factor	Bwork(+1)

TUESDAY   DATE

	Hydration (0-3) +_____	Roll(+1)
	Nutrition (0-3) +_____	Mwod(+1)
	Sleep (hrs) +_____	Stretch(+1)
	Stress (0-3)	Yoga(+1)
	Tired(0-3)	Nap(+1)
	Sore (0-3)	Msg(+1)
	Sick (0-3)	Rest(+1)
	Injured (0-3)	Ice(+1)
	Recovery Factor	Bwork(+1)

WEDNESDAY   DATE

	Hydration (0-3) +_____	Roll(+1)
	Nutrition (0-3) +_____	Mwod(+1)
	Sleep (hrs) +_____	Stretch(+1)
	Stress (0-3)	Yoga(+1)
	Tired(0-3)	Nap(+1)
	Sore (0-3)	Msg(+1)
	Sick (0-3)	Rest(+1)
	Injured (0-3)	Ice(+1)
	Recovery Factor	Bwork(+1)

THURSDAY   DATE

	Hydration (0-3) +_____	Roll(+1)
	Nutrition (0-3) +_____	Mwod(+1)
	Sleep (hrs) +_____	Stretch(+1)
	Stress (0-3)	Yoga(+1)
	Tired(0-3)	Nap(+1)
	Sore (0-3)	Msg(+1)
	Sick (0-3)	Rest(+1)
	Injured (0-3)	Ice(+1)
	Recovery Factor	Bwork(+1)

WEEKLY LOG

FRIDAY　　　　**DATE** _____

_____ Hydration (0-3) + _____ Roll(+1)
_____ Nutrition (0-3) + _____ Mwod(+1)
_____ Sleep (hrs) + _____ Stretch(+1)
_____ Stress (0-3)　　　　　　　Yoga(+1)
_____ Tired(0-3)　　　　　　　　Nap(+1)
_____ Sore (0-3)　　　　　　　　Msg(+1)
_____ Sick (0-3)　　　　　　　　Rest(+1)
_____ Injured (0-3)　　　　　　　Ice(+1)
_____ Recovery Factor　　　　　　Bwork(+1)

SATURDAY　　　　**DATE** _____

_____ Hydration (0-3) + _____ Roll(+1)
_____ Nutrition (0-3) + _____ Mwod(+1)
_____ Sleep (hrs) + _____ Stretch(+1)
_____ Stress (0-3)　　　　　　　Yoga(+1)
_____ Tired(0-3)　　　　　　　　Nap(+1)
_____ Sore (0-3)　　　　　　　　Msg(+1)
_____ Sick (0-3)　　　　　　　　Rest(+1)
_____ Injured (0-3)　　　　　　　Ice(+1)
_____ Recovery Factor　　　　　　Bwork(+1)

SUNDAY　　　　**DATE** _____

_____ Hydration (0-3) + _____ Roll(+1)
_____ Nutrition (0-3) + _____ Mwod(+1)
_____ Sleep (hrs) + _____ Stretch(+1)
_____ Stress (0-3)　　　　　　　Yoga(+1)
_____ Tired(0-3)　　　　　　　　Nap(+1)
_____ Sore (0-3)　　　　　　　　Msg(+1)
_____ Sick (0-3)　　　　　　　　Rest(+1)
_____ Injured (0-3)　　　　　　　Ice(+1)
_____ Recovery Factor　　　　　　Bwork(+1)

NOTES

Weekly RF Tracking

M _____
T _____
W _____
T _____
F _____
S _____
S _____
Average
Recovery Factor _____

BLOCK _____ CYCLE _____ WEEK _____

MONDAY   DATE _____

_____
_____
_____
_____
_____
_____
_____
_____
_____

Hydration (0-3) +_____   Roll(+1)
Nutrition (0-3) +_____   Mwod(+1)
Sleep (hrs)   +_____   Stretch(+1)
Stress (0-3)   Yoga(+1)
Tired(0-3)   Nap(+1)
Sore (0-3)   Msg(+1)
Sick (0-3)   Rest(+1)
Injured (0-3)   Ice(+1)
Recovery Factor   Bwork(+1)

TUESDAY   DATE _____

_____
_____
_____
_____
_____
_____
_____
_____
_____

Hydration (0-3) +_____   Roll(+1)
Nutrition (0-3) +_____   Mwod(+1)
Sleep (hrs)   +_____   Stretch(+1)
Stress (0-3)   Yoga(+1)
Tired(0-3)   Nap(+1)
Sore (0-3)   Msg(+1)
Sick (0-3)   Rest(+1)
Injured (0-3)   Ice(+1)
Recovery Factor   Bwork(+1)

WEDNESDAY   DATE _____

_____
_____
_____
_____
_____
_____
_____
_____
_____

Hydration (0-3) +_____   Roll(+1)
Nutrition (0-3) +_____   Mwod(+1)
Sleep (hrs)   +_____   Stretch(+1)
Stress (0-3)   Yoga(+1)
Tired(0-3)   Nap(+1)
Sore (0-3)   Msg(+1)
Sick (0-3)   Rest(+1)
Injured (0-3)   Ice(+1)
Recovery Factor   Bwork(+1)

THURSDAY   DATE _____

_____
_____
_____
_____
_____
_____
_____
_____
_____

Hydration (0-3) +_____   Roll(+1)
Nutrition (0-3) +_____   Mwod(+1)
Sleep (hrs)   +_____   Stretch(+1)
Stress (0-3)   Yoga(+1)
Tired(0-3)   Nap(+1)
Sore (0-3)   Msg(+1)
Sick (0-3)   Rest(+1)
Injured (0-3)   Ice(+1)
Recovery Factor   Bwork(+1)

WEEKLY LOG

FRIDAY   DATE _____

_____

_____

_____

_____

_____

_____

_____

_____

_____

_____

Hydration (0-3) + _____		Roll(+1)
Nutrition (0-3) + _____		Mwod(+1)
Sleep (hrs) + _____		Stretch(+1)
Stress (0-3)		Yoga(+1)
Tired(0-3)		Nap(+1)
Sore (0-3)		Msg(+1)
Sick (0-3)		Rest(+1)
Injured (0-3)		Ice(+1)
Recovery Factor		Bwork(+1)

SATURDAY   DATE _____

_____

_____

_____

_____

_____

_____

_____

_____

_____

Hydration (0-3) + _____		Roll(+1)
Nutrition (0-3) + _____		Mwod(+1)
Sleep (hrs) + _____		Stretch(+1)
Stress (0-3)		Yoga(+1)
Tired(0-3)		Nap(+1)
Sore (0-3)		Msg(+1)
Sick (0-3)		Rest(+1)
Injured (0-3)		Ice(+1)
Recovery Factor		Bwork(+1)

SUNDAY   DATE _____

_____

_____

_____

_____

_____

_____

_____

_____

_____

Hydration (0-3) + _____		Roll(+1)
Nutrition (0-3) + _____		Mwod(+1)
Sleep (hrs) + _____		Stretch(+1)
Stress (0-3)		Yoga(+1)
Tired(0-3)		Nap(+1)
Sore (0-3)		Msg(+1)
Sick (0-3)		Rest(+1)
Injured (0-3)		Ice(+1)
Recovery Factor		Bwork(+1)

NOTES

Weekly RF Tracking

M _____

T _____

W _____

T _____

F _____

S _____

S _____

Average
Recovery Factor _____

BLOCK _____ CYCLE _____ WEEK _____

MONDAY   DATE _____

_____

Hydration (0-3) +_____	Roll(+1)
Nutrition (0-3) +_____	Mwod(+1)
Sleep (hrs) +_____	Stretch(+1)
Stress (0-3)	Yoga(+1)
Tired(0-3)	Nap(+1)
Sore (0-3)	Msg(+1)
Sick (0-3)	Rest(+1)
Injured (0-3)	Ice(+1)
Recovery Factor	Bwork(+1)

TUESDAY   DATE _____

_____

Hydration (0-3) +_____	Roll(+1)
Nutrition (0-3) +_____	Mwod(+1)
Sleep (hrs) +_____	Stretch(+1)
Stress (0-3)	Yoga(+1)
Tired(0-3)	Nap(+1)
Sore (0-3)	Msg(+1)
Sick (0-3)	Rest(+1)
Injured (0-3)	Ice(+1)
Recovery Factor	Bwork(+1)

WEDNESDAY   DATE _____

_____

Hydration (0-3) +_____	Roll(+1)
Nutrition (0-3) +_____	Mwod(+1)
Sleep (hrs) +_____	Stretch(+1)
Stress (0-3)	Yoga(+1)
Tired(0-3)	Nap(+1)
Sore (0-3)	Msg(+1)
Sick (0-3)	Rest(+1)
Injured (0-3)	Ice(+1)
Recovery Factor	Bwork(+1)

THURSDAY   DATE _____

_____

Hydration (0-3) +_____	Roll(+1)
Nutrition (0-3) +_____	Mwod(+1)
Sleep (hrs) +_____	Stretch(+1)
Stress (0-3)	Yoga(+1)
Tired(0-3)	Nap(+1)
Sore (0-3)	Msg(+1)
Sick (0-3)	Rest(+1)
Injured (0-3)	Ice(+1)
Recovery Factor	Bwork(+1)

WEEKLY LOG

FRIDAY   DATE _____

_____

_____

_____

_____

_____

_____

_____

_____

_____

Hydration (0-3) + _____		Roll(+1)
Nutrition (0-3) + _____		Mwod(+1)
Sleep (hrs) + _____		Stretch(+1)
Stress (0-3)		Yoga(+1)
Tired(0-3)		Nap(+1)
Sore (0-3)		Msg(+1)
Sick (0-3)		Rest(+1)
Injured (0-3)		Ice(+1)
Recovery Factor		Bwork(+1)

SATURDAY   DATE _____

_____

_____

_____

_____

_____

_____

_____

_____

_____

Hydration (0-3) + _____		Roll(+1)
Nutrition (0-3) + _____		Mwod(+1)
Sleep (hrs) + _____		Stretch(+1)
Stress (0-3)		Yoga(+1)
Tired(0-3)		Nap(+1)
Sore (0-3)		Msg(+1)
Sick (0-3)		Rest(+1)
Injured (0-3)		Ice(+1)
Recovery Factor		Bwork(+1)

SUNDAY   DATE _____

_____

_____

_____

_____

_____

_____

_____

_____

_____

Hydration (0-3) + _____		Roll(+1)
Nutrition (0-3) + _____		Mwod(+1)
Sleep (hrs) + _____		Stretch(+1)
Stress (0-3)		Yoga(+1)
Tired(0-3)		Nap(+1)
Sore (0-3)		Msg(+1)
Sick (0-3)		Rest(+1)
Injured (0-3)		Ice(+1)
Recovery Factor		Bwork(+1)

NOTES

Weekly RF Tracking

M _____

T _____

W _____

T _____

F _____

S _____

S _____

Average
Recovery Factor _____

BLOCK _____ CYCLE _____ WEEK _____

MONDAY   DATE

_____
_____
_____
_____
_____
_____
_____
_____

Hydration (0-3) +_____ Roll(+1)
Nutrition (0-3) +_____ Mwod(+1)
Sleep (hrs) +_____ Stretch(+1)
Stress (0-3) Yoga(+1)
Tired(0-3) Nap(+1)
Sore (0-3) Msg(+1)
Sick (0-3) Rest(+1)
Injured (0-3) Ice(+1)
Recovery Factor Bwork(+1)

TUESDAY   DATE

_____
_____
_____
_____
_____
_____
_____
_____

Hydration (0-3) +_____ Roll(+1)
Nutrition (0-3) +_____ Mwod(+1)
Sleep (hrs) +_____ Stretch(+1)
Stress (0-3) Yoga(+1)
Tired(0-3) Nap(+1)
Sore (0-3) Msg(+1)
Sick (0-3) Rest(+1)
Injured (0-3) Ice(+1)
Recovery Factor Bwork(+1)

WEDNESDAY   DATE

_____
_____
_____
_____
_____
_____
_____
_____

Hydration (0-3) +_____ Roll(+1)
Nutrition (0-3) +_____ Mwod(+1)
Sleep (hrs) +_____ Stretch(+1)
Stress (0-3) Yoga(+1)
Tired(0-3) Nap(+1)
Sore (0-3) Msg(+1)
Sick (0-3) Rest(+1)
Injured (0-3) Ice(+1)
Recovery Factor Bwork(+1)

THURSDAY   DATE

_____
_____
_____
_____
_____
_____
_____
_____

Hydration (0-3) +_____ Roll(+1)
Nutrition (0-3) +_____ Mwod(+1)
Sleep (hrs) +_____ Stretch(+1)
Stress (0-3) Yoga(+1)
Tired(0-3) Nap(+1)
Sore (0-3) Msg(+1)
Sick (0-3) Rest(+1)
Injured (0-3) Ice(+1)
Recovery Factor Bwork(+1)

WEEKLY LOG

FRIDAY   **DATE**

_____
_____
_____
_____
_____
_____
_____
_____
_____

Hydration (0-3) +_____ Roll(+1)
Nutrition (0-3) +_____ Mwod(+1)
Sleep (hrs)   +_____ Stretch(+1)
Stress (0-3)   Yoga(+1)
Tired(0-3)   Nap(+1)
Sore (0-3)   Msg(+1)
Sick (0-3)   Rest(+1)
Injured (0-3)   Ice(+1)
Recovery Factor   Bwork(+1)

SATURDAY   **DATE**

_____
_____
_____
_____
_____
_____
_____
_____
_____

Hydration (0-3) +_____ Roll(+1)
Nutrition (0-3) +_____ Mwod(+1)
Sleep (hrs)   +_____ Stretch(+1)
Stress (0-3)   Yoga(+1)
Tired(0-3)   Nap(+1)
Sore (0-3)   Msg(+1)
Sick (0-3)   Rest(+1)
Injured (0-3)   Ice(+1)
Recovery Factor   Bwork(+1)

SUNDAY   **DATE**

_____
_____
_____
_____
_____
_____
_____
_____
_____

Hydration (0-3) +_____ Roll(+1)
Nutrition (0-3) +_____ Mwod(+1)
Sleep (hrs)   +_____ Stretch(+1)
Stress (0-3)   Yoga(+1)
Tired(0-3)   Nap(+1)
Sore (0-3)   Msg(+1)
Sick (0-3)   Rest(+1)
Injured (0-3)   Ice(+1)
Recovery Factor   Bwork(+1)

NOTES

Weekly RF Tracking

M _____
T _____
W _____
T _____
F _____
S _____
S _____
Average
Recovery Factor _____

BLOCK _____ CYCLE _____ WEEK _____

MONDAY   DATE _____

_____

_____

_____

_____

_____

_____

_____

_____

_____

Hydration (0-3) +_____	Roll(+1)
Nutrition (0-3) +_____	Mwod(+1)
Sleep (hrs) +_____	Stretch(+1)
Stress (0-3)	Yoga(+1)
Tired(0-3)	Nap(+1)
Sore (0-3)	Msg(+1)
Sick (0-3)	Rest(+1)
Injured (0-3)	Ice(+1)
Recovery Factor	Bwork(+1)

TUESDAY   DATE _____

_____

_____

_____

_____

_____

_____

_____

_____

_____

Hydration (0-3) +_____	Roll(+1)
Nutrition (0-3) +_____	Mwod(+1)
Sleep (hrs) +_____	Stretch(+1)
Stress (0-3)	Yoga(+1)
Tired(0-3)	Nap(+1)
Sore (0-3)	Msg(+1)
Sick (0-3)	Rest(+1)
Injured (0-3)	Ice(+1)
Recovery Factor	Bwork(+1)

WEDNESDAY   DATE _____

_____

_____

_____

_____

_____

_____

_____

_____

_____

Hydration (0-3) +_____	Roll(+1)
Nutrition (0-3) +_____	Mwod(+1)
Sleep (hrs) +_____	Stretch(+1)
Stress (0-3)	Yoga(+1)
Tired(0-3)	Nap(+1)
Sore (0-3)	Msg(+1)
Sick (0-3)	Rest(+1)
Injured (0-3)	Ice(+1)
Recovery Factor	Bwork(+1)

THURSDAY   DATE _____

_____

_____

_____

_____

_____

_____

_____

_____

_____

Hydration (0-3) +_____	Roll(+1)
Nutrition (0-3) +_____	Mwod(+1)
Sleep (hrs) +_____	Stretch(+1)
Stress (0-3)	Yoga(+1)
Tired(0-3)	Nap(+1)
Sore (0-3)	Msg(+1)
Sick (0-3)	Rest(+1)
Injured (0-3)	Ice(+1)
Recovery Factor	Bwork(+1)

WEEKLY LOG

FRIDAY   DATE _____

_____ Hydration (0-3) +_____ Roll(+1)
_____ Nutrition (0-3) +_____ Mwod(+1)
_____ Sleep (hrs)   +_____ Stretch(+1)
_____ Stress (0-3)   Yoga(+1)
_____ Tired(0-3)   Nap(+1)
_____ Sore (0-3)   Msg(+1)
_____ Sick (0-3)   Rest(+1)
_____ Injured (0-3)   Ice(+1)
_____ Recovery Factor   Bwork(+1)

SATURDAY   DATE _____

_____ Hydration (0-3) +_____ Roll(+1)
_____ Nutrition (0-3) +_____ Mwod(+1)
_____ Sleep (hrs)   +_____ Stretch(+1)
_____ Stress (0-3)   Yoga(+1)
_____ Tired(0-3)   Nap(+1)
_____ Sore (0-3)   Msg(+1)
_____ Sick (0-3)   Rest(+1)
_____ Injured (0-3)   Ice(+1)
_____ Recovery Factor   Bwork(+1)

SUNDAY   DATE _____

_____ Hydration (0-3) +_____ Roll(+1)
_____ Nutrition (0-3) +_____ Mwod(+1)
_____ Sleep (hrs)   +_____ Stretch(+1)
_____ Stress (0-3)   Yoga(+1)
_____ Tired(0-3)   Nap(+1)
_____ Sore (0-3)   Msg(+1)
_____ Sick (0-3)   Rest(+1)
_____ Injured (0-3)   Ice(+1)
_____ Recovery Factor   Bwork(+1)

NOTES

Weekly RF Tracking

M _____
T _____
W _____
T _____
F _____
S _____
S _____
Average
Recovery Factor _____

BLOCK _____ CYCLE _____ WEEK _____

MONDAY   DATE

_____   Hydration (0-3) + _____   Roll(+1)
_____   Nutrition (0-3) + _____   Mwod(+1)
_____   Sleep (hrs)   + _____   Stretch(+1)
_____   Stress (0-3)   Yoga(+1)
_____   Tired(0-3)   Nap(+1)
_____   Sore (0-3)   Msg(+1)
_____   Sick (0-3)   Rest(+1)
_____   Injured (0-3)   Ice(+1)
_____   Recovery Factor   Bwork(+1)

TUESDAY   DATE

_____   Hydration (0-3) + _____   Roll(+1)
_____   Nutrition (0-3) + _____   Mwod(+1)
_____   Sleep (hrs)   + _____   Stretch(+1)
_____   Stress (0-3)   Yoga(+1)
_____   Tired(0-3)   Nap(+1)
_____   Sore (0-3)   Msg(+1)
_____   Sick (0-3)   Rest(+1)
_____   Injured (0-3)   Ice(+1)
_____   Recovery Factor   Bwork(+1)

WEDNESDAY   DATE

_____   Hydration (0-3) + _____   Roll(+1)
_____   Nutrition (0-3) + _____   Mwod(+1)
_____   Sleep (hrs)   + _____   Stretch(+1)
_____   Stress (0-3)   Yoga(+1)
_____   Tired(0-3)   Nap(+1)
_____   Sore (0-3)   Msg(+1)
_____   Sick (0-3)   Rest(+1)
_____   Injured (0-3)   Ice(+1)
_____   Recovery Factor   Bwork(+1)

THURSDAY   DATE

_____   Hydration (0-3) + _____   Roll(+1)
_____   Nutrition (0-3) + _____   Mwod(+1)
_____   Sleep (hrs)   + _____   Stretch(+1)
_____   Stress (0-3)   Yoga(+1)
_____   Tired(0-3)   Nap(+1)
_____   Sore (0-3)   Msg(+1)
_____   Sick (0-3)   Rest(+1)
_____   Injured (0-3)   Ice(+1)
_____   Recovery Factor   Bwork(+1)

WEEKLY LOG

FRIDAY   DATE _____

_____

_____

_____

_____

_____

_____

_____

_____

Hydration (0-3) + _____		Roll(+1)
Nutrition (0-3) + _____		Mwod(+1)
Sleep (hrs) + _____		Stretch(+1)
Stress (0-3)		Yoga(+1)
Tired(0-3)		Nap(+1)
Sore (0-3)		Msg(+1)
Sick (0-3)		Rest(+1)
Injured (0-3)		Ice(+1)
Recovery Factor		Bwork(+1)

SATURDAY   DATE _____

_____

_____

_____

_____

_____

_____

_____

_____

Hydration (0-3) + _____		Roll(+1)
Nutrition (0-3) + _____		Mwod(+1)
Sleep (hrs) + _____		Stretch(+1)
Stress (0-3)		Yoga(+1)
Tired(0-3)		Nap(+1)
Sore (0-3)		Msg(+1)
Sick (0-3)		Rest(+1)
Injured (0-3)		Ice(+1)
Recovery Factor		Bwork(+1)

SUNDAY   DATE _____

_____

_____

_____

_____

_____

_____

_____

_____

Hydration (0-3) + _____		Roll(+1)
Nutrition (0-3) + _____		Mwod(+1)
Sleep (hrs) + _____		Stretch(+1)
Stress (0-3)		Yoga(+1)
Tired(0-3)		Nap(+1)
Sore (0-3)		Msg(+1)
Sick (0-3)		Rest(+1)
Injured (0-3)		Ice(+1)
Recovery Factor		Bwork(+1)

NOTES

Weekly RF Tracking

M _____

T _____

W _____

T _____

F _____

S _____

S _____

Average
Recovery Factor _____

BLOCK _____ CYCLE _____ WEEK _____

MONDAY   DATE

_____

_____

_____

_____

_____

_____

_____

Hydration (0-3) +	_____	Roll(+1)
Nutrition (0-3) +	_____	Mwod(+1)
Sleep (hrs) +	_____	Stretch(+1)
Stress (0-3)		Yoga(+1)
Tired(0-3)		Nap(+1)
Sore (0-3)		Msg(+1)
Sick (0-3)		Rest(+1)
Injured (0-3)		Ice(+1)
Recovery Factor		Bwork(+1)

TUESDAY   DATE

_____

_____

_____

_____

_____

_____

_____

Hydration (0-3) +	_____	Roll(+1)
Nutrition (0-3) +	_____	Mwod(+1)
Sleep (hrs) +	_____	Stretch(+1)
Stress (0-3)		Yoga(+1)
Tired(0-3)		Nap(+1)
Sore (0-3)		Msg(+1)
Sick (0-3)		Rest(+1)
Injured (0-3)		Ice(+1)
Recovery Factor		Bwork(+1)

WEDNESDAY   DATE

_____

_____

_____

_____

_____

_____

_____

Hydration (0-3) +	_____	Roll(+1)
Nutrition (0-3) +	_____	Mwod(+1)
Sleep (hrs) +	_____	Stretch(+1)
Stress (0-3)		Yoga(+1)
Tired(0-3)		Nap(+1)
Sore (0-3)		Msg(+1)
Sick (0-3)		Rest(+1)
Injured (0-3)		Ice(+1)
Recovery Factor		Bwork(+1)

THURSDAY   DATE

_____

_____

_____

_____

_____

_____

_____

Hydration (0-3) +	_____	Roll(+1)
Nutrition (0-3) +	_____	Mwod(+1)
Sleep (hrs) +	_____	Stretch(+1)
Stress (0-3)		Yoga(+1)
Tired(0-3)		Nap(+1)
Sore (0-3)		Msg(+1)
Sick (0-3)		Rest(+1)
Injured (0-3)		Ice(+1)
Recovery Factor		Bwork(+1)

WEEKLY LOG

FRIDAY   **DATE** _____

_____

_____

_____

_____

_____

_____

_____

_____

Hydration (0-3) +_____	Roll(+1)
Nutrition (0-3) +_____	Mwod(+1)
Sleep (hrs) +_____	Stretch(+1)
Stress (0-3)	Yoga(+1)
Tired(0-3)	Nap(+1)
Sore (0-3)	Msg(+1)
Sick (0-3)	Rest(+1)
Injured (0-3)	Ice(+1)
Recovery Factor	Bwork(+1)

SATURDAY   **DATE** _____

_____

_____

_____

_____

_____

_____

_____

_____

Hydration (0-3) +_____	Roll(+1)
Nutrition (0-3) +_____	Mwod(+1)
Sleep (hrs) +_____	Stretch(+1)
Stress (0-3)	Yoga(+1)
Tired(0-3)	Nap(+1)
Sore (0-3)	Msg(+1)
Sick (0-3)	Rest(+1)
Injured (0-3)	Ice(+1)
Recovery Factor	Bwork(+1)

SUNDAY   **DATE** _____

_____

_____

_____

_____

_____

_____

_____

_____

Hydration (0-3) +_____	Roll(+1)
Nutrition (0-3) +_____	Mwod(+1)
Sleep (hrs) +_____	Stretch(+1)
Stress (0-3)	Yoga(+1)
Tired(0-3)	Nap(+1)
Sore (0-3)	Msg(+1)
Sick (0-3)	Rest(+1)
Injured (0-3)	Ice(+1)
Recovery Factor	Bwork(+1)

NOTES

Weekly RF Tracking

M _____

T _____

W _____

T _____

F _____

S _____

S _____

Average
Recovery Factor _____

BLOCK _____ CYCLE _____ WEEK _____

MONDAY _____ DATE _____

_____

Hydration (0-3) + _____	Roll(+1)
Nutrition (0-3) + _____	Mwod(+1)
Sleep (hrs) + _____	Stretch(+1)
Stress (0-3)	Yoga(+1)
Tired(0-3)	Nap(+1)
Sore (0-3)	Msg(+1)
Sick (0-3)	Rest(+1)
Injured (0-3)	Ice(+1)
Recovery Factor	Bwork(+1)

TUESDAY _____ DATE _____

_____

Hydration (0-3) + _____	Roll(+1)
Nutrition (0-3) + _____	Mwod(+1)
Sleep (hrs) + _____	Stretch(+1)
Stress (0-3)	Yoga(+1)
Tired(0-3)	Nap(+1)
Sore (0-3)	Msg(+1)
Sick (0-3)	Rest(+1)
Injured (0-3)	Ice(+1)
Recovery Factor	Bwork(+1)

WEDNESDAY _____ DATE _____

_____

Hydration (0-3) + _____	Roll(+1)
Nutrition (0-3) + _____	Mwod(+1)
Sleep (hrs) + _____	Stretch(+1)
Stress (0-3)	Yoga(+1)
Tired(0-3)	Nap(+1)
Sore (0-3)	Msg(+1)
Sick (0-3)	Rest(+1)
Injured (0-3)	Ice(+1)
Recovery Factor	Bwork(+1)

THURSDAY _____ DATE _____

_____

Hydration (0-3) + _____	Roll(+1)
Nutrition (0-3) + _____	Mwod(+1)
Sleep (hrs) + _____	Stretch(+1)
Stress (0-3)	Yoga(+1)
Tired(0-3)	Nap(+1)
Sore (0-3)	Msg(+1)
Sick (0-3)	Rest(+1)
Injured (0-3)	Ice(+1)
Recovery Factor	Bwork(+1)

WEEKLY LOG

FRIDAY   DATE

_____

Hydration (0-3) +_____ Roll(+1)

Nutrition (0-3) +_____ Mwod(+1)

Sleep (hrs) +_____ Stretch(+1)

Stress (0-3)   Yoga(+1)

Tired(0-3)   Nap(+1)

Sore (0-3)   Msg(+1)

Sick (0-3)   Rest(+1)

Injured (0-3)   Ice(+1)

Recovery Factor   Bwork(+1)

SATURDAY   DATE

_____

Hydration (0-3) +_____ Roll(+1)

Nutrition (0-3) +_____ Mwod(+1)

Sleep (hrs) +_____ Stretch(+1)

Stress (0-3)   Yoga(+1)

Tired(0-3)   Nap(+1)

Sore (0-3)   Msg(+1)

Sick (0-3)   Rest(+1)

Injured (0-3)   Ice(+1)

Recovery Factor   Bwork(+1)

SUNDAY   DATE

_____

Hydration (0-3) +_____ Roll(+1)

Nutrition (0-3) +_____ Mwod(+1)

Sleep (hrs) +_____ Stretch(+1)

Stress (0-3)   Yoga(+1)

Tired(0-3)   Nap(+1)

Sore (0-3)   Msg(+1)

Sick (0-3)   Rest(+1)

Injured (0-3)   Ice(+1)

Recovery Factor   Bwork(+1)

NOTES

Weekly RF Tracking

M _____

T _____

W _____

T _____

F _____

S _____

S _____

Average
Recovery Factor _____

BLOCK _____ CYCLE _____ WEEK _____

MONDAY   DATE

Hydration (0-3) +_____	Roll(+1)
Nutrition (0-3) +_____	Mwod(+1)
Sleep (hrs) +_____	Stretch(+1)
Stress (0-3)	Yoga(+1)
Tired(0-3)	Nap(+1)
Sore (0-3)	Msg(+1)
Sick (0-3)	Rest(+1)
Injured (0-3)	Ice(+1)
Recovery Factor	Bwork(+1)

TUESDAY   DATE

Hydration (0-3) +_____	Roll(+1)
Nutrition (0-3) +_____	Mwod(+1)
Sleep (hrs) +_____	Stretch(+1)
Stress (0-3)	Yoga(+1)
Tired(0-3)	Nap(+1)
Sore (0-3)	Msg(+1)
Sick (0-3)	Rest(+1)
Injured (0-3)	Ice(+1)
Recovery Factor	Bwork(+1)

WEDNESDAY   DATE

Hydration (0-3) +_____	Roll(+1)
Nutrition (0-3) +_____	Mwod(+1)
Sleep (hrs) +_____	Stretch(+1)
Stress (0-3)	Yoga(+1)
Tired(0-3)	Nap(+1)
Sore (0-3)	Msg(+1)
Sick (0-3)	Rest(+1)
Injured (0-3)	Ice(+1)
Recovery Factor	Bwork(+1)

THURSDAY   DATE

Hydration (0-3) +_____	Roll(+1)
Nutrition (0-3) +_____	Mwod(+1)
Sleep (hrs) +_____	Stretch(+1)
Stress (0-3)	Yoga(+1)
Tired(0-3)	Nap(+1)
Sore (0-3)	Msg(+1)
Sick (0-3)	Rest(+1)
Injured (0-3)	Ice(+1)
Recovery Factor	Bwork(+1)

WEEKLY LOG

FRIDAY   DATE

_____

Hydration (0-3) +_____	Roll(+1)
Nutrition (0-3) +_____	Mwod(+1)
Sleep (hrs) +_____	Stretch(+1)
Stress (0-3)	Yoga(+1)
Tired(0-3)	Nap(+1)
Sore (0-3)	Msg(+1)
Sick (0-3)	Rest(+1)
Injured (0-3)	Ice(+1)
Recovery Factor	Bwork(+1)

SATURDAY   DATE

_____

Hydration (0-3) +_____	Roll(+1)
Nutrition (0-3) +_____	Mwod(+1)
Sleep (hrs) +_____	Stretch(+1)
Stress (0-3)	Yoga(+1)
Tired(0-3)	Nap(+1)
Sore (0-3)	Msg(+1)
Sick (0-3)	Rest(+1)
Injured (0-3)	Ice(+1)
Recovery Factor	Bwork(+1)

SUNDAY   DATE

_____

Hydration (0-3) +_____	Roll(+1)
Nutrition (0-3) +_____	Mwod(+1)
Sleep (hrs) +_____	Stretch(+1)
Stress (0-3)	Yoga(+1)
Tired(0-3)	Nap(+1)
Sore (0-3)	Msg(+1)
Sick (0-3)	Rest(+1)
Injured (0-3)	Ice(+1)
Recovery Factor	Bwork(+1)

NOTES

Weekly RF Tracking

M _____
T _____
W _____
T _____
F _____
S _____
S _____
Average
Recovery Factor _____

BLOCK _____ CYCLE _____ WEEK _____

MONDAY   DATE

Hydration (0-3) +_____	Roll(+1)
Nutrition (0-3) +_____	Mwod(+1)
Sleep (hrs) +_____	Stretch(+1)
Stress (0-3)	Yoga(+1)
Tired(0-3)	Nap(+1)
Sore (0-3)	Msg(+1)
Sick (0-3)	Rest(+1)
Injured (0-3)	Ice(+1)
Recovery Factor	Bwork(+1)

TUESDAY   DATE

Hydration (0-3) +_____	Roll(+1)
Nutrition (0-3) +_____	Mwod(+1)
Sleep (hrs) +_____	Stretch(+1)
Stress (0-3)	Yoga(+1)
Tired(0-3)	Nap(+1)
Sore (0-3)	Msg(+1)
Sick (0-3)	Rest(+1)
Injured (0-3)	Ice(+1)
Recovery Factor	Bwork(+1)

WEDNESDAY   DATE

Hydration (0-3) +_____	Roll(+1)
Nutrition (0-3) +_____	Mwod(+1)
Sleep (hrs) +_____	Stretch(+1)
Stress (0-3)	Yoga(+1)
Tired(0-3)	Nap(+1)
Sore (0-3)	Msg(+1)
Sick (0-3)	Rest(+1)
Injured (0-3)	Ice(+1)
Recovery Factor	Bwork(+1)

THURSDAY   DATE

Hydration (0-3) +_____	Roll(+1)
Nutrition (0-3) +_____	Mwod(+1)
Sleep (hrs) +_____	Stretch(+1)
Stress (0-3)	Yoga(+1)
Tired(0-3)	Nap(+1)
Sore (0-3)	Msg(+1)
Sick (0-3)	Rest(+1)
Injured (0-3)	Ice(+1)
Recovery Factor	Bwork(+1)

WEEKLY LOG

FRIDAY   **DATE** _____

_____

_____

_____

_____

_____

_____

_____

_____

Hydration (0-3)	+_____	Roll(+1)
Nutrition (0-3)	+_____	Mwod(+1)
Sleep (hrs)	+_____	Stretch(+1)
Stress (0-3)		Yoga(+1)
Tired(0-3)		Nap(+1)
Sore (0-3)		Msg(+1)
Sick (0-3)		Rest(+1)
Injured (0-3)		Ice(+1)
Recovery Factor		Bwork(+1)

SATURDAY   **DATE** _____

_____

_____

_____

_____

_____

_____

_____

_____

Hydration (0-3)	+_____	Roll(+1)
Nutrition (0-3)	+_____	Mwod(+1)
Sleep (hrs)	+_____	Stretch(+1)
Stress (0-3)		Yoga(+1)
Tired(0-3)		Nap(+1)
Sore (0-3)		Msg(+1)
Sick (0-3)		Rest(+1)
Injured (0-3)		Ice(+1)
Recovery Factor		Bwork(+1)

SUNDAY   **DATE** _____

_____

_____

_____

_____

_____

_____

_____

_____

Hydration (0-3)	+_____	Roll(+1)
Nutrition (0-3)	+_____	Mwod(+1)
Sleep (hrs)	+_____	Stretch(+1)
Stress (0-3)		Yoga(+1)
Tired(0-3)		Nap(+1)
Sore (0-3)		Msg(+1)
Sick (0-3)		Rest(+1)
Injured (0-3)		Ice(+1)
Recovery Factor		Bwork(+1)

NOTES

Weekly RF Tracking

M _____

T _____

W _____

T _____

F _____

S _____

S _____

Average
Recovery Factor _____

BLOCK _____ CYCLE _____ WEEK _____

MONDAY _____ DATE _____

Hydration (0-3) +_____	Roll(+1)
Nutrition (0-3) +_____	Mwod(+1)
Sleep (hrs) +_____	Stretch(+1)
Stress (0-3)	Yoga(+1)
Tired(0-3)	Nap(+1)
Sore (0-3)	Msg(+1)
Sick (0-3)	Rest(+1)
Injured (0-3)	Ice(+1)
Recovery Factor	Bwork(+1)

TUESDAY _____ DATE _____

Hydration (0-3) +_____	Roll(+1)
Nutrition (0-3) +_____	Mwod(+1)
Sleep (hrs) +_____	Stretch(+1)
Stress (0-3)	Yoga(+1)
Tired(0-3)	Nap(+1)
Sore (0-3)	Msg(+1)
Sick (0-3)	Rest(+1)
Injured (0-3)	Ice(+1)
Recovery Factor	Bwork(+1)

WEDNESDAY _____ DATE _____

Hydration (0-3) +_____	Roll(+1)
Nutrition (0-3) +_____	Mwod(+1)
Sleep (hrs) +_____	Stretch(+1)
Stress (0-3)	Yoga(+1)
Tired(0-3)	Nap(+1)
Sore (0-3)	Msg(+1)
Sick (0-3)	Rest(+1)
Injured (0-3)	Ice(+1)
Recovery Factor	Bwork(+1)

THURSDAY _____ DATE _____

Hydration (0-3) +_____	Roll(+1)
Nutrition (0-3) +_____	Mwod(+1)
Sleep (hrs) +_____	Stretch(+1)
Stress (0-3)	Yoga(+1)
Tired(0-3)	Nap(+1)
Sore (0-3)	Msg(+1)
Sick (0-3)	Rest(+1)
Injured (0-3)	Ice(+1)
Recovery Factor	Bwork(+1)

WEEKLY LOG

FRIDAY   DATE _____

_____   Hydration (0-3) +_____ Roll(+1)
_____   Nutrition (0-3) +_____ Mwod(+1)
_____   Sleep (hrs)   +_____ Stretch(+1)
_____   Stress (0-3)   Yoga(+1)
_____   Tired(0-3)   Nap(+1)
_____   Sore (0-3)   Msg(+1)
_____   Sick (0-3)   Rest(+1)
_____   Injured (0-3)   Ice(+1)
_____   Recovery Factor   Bwork(+1)

SATURDAY   DATE _____

_____   Hydration (0-3) +_____ Roll(+1)
_____   Nutrition (0-3) +_____ Mwod(+1)
_____   Sleep (hrs)   +_____ Stretch(+1)
_____   Stress (0-3)   Yoga(+1)
_____   Tired(0-3)   Nap(+1)
_____   Sore (0-3)   Msg(+1)
_____   Sick (0-3)   Rest(+1)
_____   Injured (0-3)   Ice(+1)
_____   Recovery Factor   Bwork(+1)

SUNDAY   DATE _____

_____   Hydration (0-3) +_____ Roll(+1)
_____   Nutrition (0-3) +_____ Mwod(+1)
_____   Sleep (hrs)   +_____ Stretch(+1)
_____   Stress (0-3)   Yoga(+1)
_____   Tired(0-3)   Nap(+1)
_____   Sore (0-3)   Msg(+1)
_____   Sick (0-3)   Rest(+1)
_____   Injured (0-3)   Ice(+1)
_____   Recovery Factor   Bwork(+1)

NOTES

Weekly RF Tracking

M _____
T _____
W _____
T _____
F _____
S _____
S _____
Average
Recovery Factor _____

BLOCK _____ CYCLE _____ WEEK _____

MONDAY _____ DATE _____

_____

Hydration (0-3) +_____		Roll(+1)
Nutrition (0-3) +_____		Mwod(+1)
Sleep (hrs) +_____		Stretch(+1)
Stress (0-3)		Yoga(+1)
Tired(0-3)		Nap(+1)
Sore (0-3)		Msg(+1)
Sick (0-3)		Rest(+1)
Injured (0-3)		Ice(+1)
Recovery Factor		Bwork(+1)

TUESDAY _____ DATE _____

_____

Hydration (0-3) +_____		Roll(+1)
Nutrition (0-3) +_____		Mwod(+1)
Sleep (hrs) +_____		Stretch(+1)
Stress (0-3)		Yoga(+1)
Tired(0-3)		Nap(+1)
Sore (0-3)		Msg(+1)
Sick (0-3)		Rest(+1)
Injured (0-3)		Ice(+1)
Recovery Factor		Bwork(+1)

WEDNESDAY _____ DATE _____

_____

Hydration (0-3) +_____		Roll(+1)
Nutrition (0-3) +_____		Mwod(+1)
Sleep (hrs) +_____		Stretch(+1)
Stress (0-3)		Yoga(+1)
Tired(0-3)		Nap(+1)
Sore (0-3)		Msg(+1)
Sick (0-3)		Rest(+1)
Injured (0-3)		Ice(+1)
Recovery Factor		Bwork(+1)

THURSDAY _____ DATE _____

_____

Hydration (0-3) +_____		Roll(+1)
Nutrition (0-3) +_____		Mwod(+1)
Sleep (hrs) +_____		Stretch(+1)
Stress (0-3)		Yoga(+1)
Tired(0-3)		Nap(+1)
Sore (0-3)		Msg(+1)
Sick (0-3)		Rest(+1)
Injured (0-3)		Ice(+1)
Recovery Factor		Bwork(+1)

WEEKLY LOG

FRIDAY   DATE

_____

_____

_____

_____

_____

_____

_____

_____

Hydration (0-3) +	_____	Roll(+1)
Nutrition (0-3) +	_____	Mwod(+1)
Sleep (hrs) +	_____	Stretch(+1)
Stress (0-3)		Yoga(+1)
Tired(0-3)		Nap(+1)
Sore (0-3)		Msg(+1)
Sick (0-3)		Rest(+1)
Injured (0-3)		Ice(+1)
Recovery Factor		Bwork(+1)

SATURDAY   DATE

_____

_____

_____

_____

_____

_____

_____

_____

Hydration (0-3) +	_____	Roll(+1)
Nutrition (0-3) +	_____	Mwod(+1)
Sleep (hrs) +	_____	Stretch(+1)
Stress (0-3)		Yoga(+1)
Tired(0-3)		Nap(+1)
Sore (0-3)		Msg(+1)
Sick (0-3)		Rest(+1)
Injured (0-3)		Ice(+1)
Recovery Factor		Bwork(+1)

SUNDAY   DATE

_____

_____

_____

_____

_____

_____

_____

_____

Hydration (0-3) +	_____	Roll(+1)
Nutrition (0-3) +	_____	Mwod(+1)
Sleep (hrs) +	_____	Stretch(+1)
Stress (0-3)		Yoga(+1)
Tired(0-3)		Nap(+1)
Sore (0-3)		Msg(+1)
Sick (0-3)		Rest(+1)
Injured (0-3)		Ice(+1)
Recovery Factor		Bwork(+1)

NOTES

Weekly RF Tracking

M _____

T _____

W _____

T _____

F _____

S _____

S _____

Average
Recovery Factor _____

BLOCK _____ CYCLE _____ WEEK _____

MONDAY   DATE _____

_____

_____

_____

_____

_____

_____

_____

_____

Hydration (0-3) + _____	Roll(+1)
Nutrition (0-3) + _____	Mwod(+1)
Sleep (hrs) + _____	Stretch(+1)
Stress (0-3)	Yoga(+1)
Tired(0-3)	Nap(+1)
Sore (0-3)	Msg(+1)
Sick (0-3)	Rest(+1)
Injured (0-3)	Ice(+1)
Recovery Factor	Bwork(+1)

TUESDAY   DATE _____

_____

_____

_____

_____

_____

_____

_____

_____

Hydration (0-3) + _____	Roll(+1)
Nutrition (0-3) + _____	Mwod(+1)
Sleep (hrs) + _____	Stretch(+1)
Stress (0-3)	Yoga(+1)
Tired(0-3)	Nap(+1)
Sore (0-3)	Msg(+1)
Sick (0-3)	Rest(+1)
Injured (0-3)	Ice(+1)
Recovery Factor	Bwork(+1)

WEDNESDAY   DATE _____

_____

_____

_____

_____

_____

_____

_____

_____

Hydration (0-3) + _____	Roll(+1)
Nutrition (0-3) + _____	Mwod(+1)
Sleep (hrs) + _____	Stretch(+1)
Stress (0-3)	Yoga(+1)
Tired(0-3)	Nap(+1)
Sore (0-3)	Msg(+1)
Sick (0-3)	Rest(+1)
Injured (0-3)	Ice(+1)
Recovery Factor	Bwork(+1)

THURSDAY   DATE _____

_____

_____

_____

_____

_____

_____

_____

_____

Hydration (0-3) + _____	Roll(+1)
Nutrition (0-3) + _____	Mwod(+1)
Sleep (hrs) + _____	Stretch(+1)
Stress (0-3)	Yoga(+1)
Tired(0-3)	Nap(+1)
Sore (0-3)	Msg(+1)
Sick (0-3)	Rest(+1)
Injured (0-3)	Ice(+1)
Recovery Factor	Bwork(+1)

WEEKLY LOG

FRIDAY   DATE

_____

Hydration (0-3) + _____		Roll(+1)
Nutrition (0-3) + _____		Mwod(+1)
Sleep (hrs) + _____		Stretch(+1)
Stress (0-3)	-	Yoga(+1)
Tired(0-3)	-	Nap(+1)
Sore (0-3)	-	Msg(+1)
Sick (0-3)	-	Rest(+1)
Injured (0-3)	-	Ice(+1)
Recovery Factor		Bwork(+1)

SATURDAY   DATE

_____

Hydration (0-3) + _____		Roll(+1)
Nutrition (0-3) + _____		Mwod(+1)
Sleep (hrs) + _____		Stretch(+1)
Stress (0-3)	-	Yoga(+1)
Tired(0-3)	-	Nap(+1)
Sore (0-3)	-	Msg(+1)
Sick (0-3)	-	Rest(+1)
Injured (0-3)	-	Ice(+1)
Recovery Factor		Bwork(+1)

SUNDAY   DATE

_____

Hydration (0-3) + _____		Roll(+1)
Nutrition (0-3) + _____		Mwod(+1)
Sleep (hrs) + _____		Stretch(+1)
Stress (0-3)	-	Yoga(+1)
Tired(0-3)	-	Nap(+1)
Sore (0-3)	-	Msg(+1)
Sick (0-3)	-	Rest(+1)
Injured (0-3)	-	Ice(+1)
Recovery Factor		Bwork(+1)

NOTES

Weekly RF Tracking

M _____
T _____
W _____
T _____
F _____
S _____
S _____

Average
Recovery Factor _____

BLOCK _____ CYCLE _____ WEEK _____

MONDAY   DATE

_____ Hydration (0-3) +_____ Roll(+1)
_____ Nutrition (0-3) +_____ Mwod(+1)
_____ Sleep (hrs)   +_____ Stretch(+1)
_____ Stress (0-3)   Yoga(+1)
_____ Tired(0-3)   Nap(+1)
_____ Sore (0-3)   Msg(+1)
_____ Sick (0-3)   Rest(+1)
_____ Injured (0-3)   Ice(+1)
_____ Recovery Factor   Bwork(+1)

TUESDAY   DATE

_____ Hydration (0-3) +_____ Roll(+1)
_____ Nutrition (0-3) +_____ Mwod(+1)
_____ Sleep (hrs)   +_____ Stretch(+1)
_____ Stress (0-3)   Yoga(+1)
_____ Tired(0-3)   Nap(+1)
_____ Sore (0-3)   Msg(+1)
_____ Sick (0-3)   Rest(+1)
_____ Injured (0-3)   Ice(+1)
_____ Recovery Factor   Bwork(+1)

WEDNESDAY   DATE

_____ Hydration (0-3) +_____ Roll(+1)
_____ Nutrition (0-3) +_____ Mwod(+1)
_____ Sleep (hrs)   +_____ Stretch(+1)
_____ Stress (0-3)   Yoga(+1)
_____ Tired(0-3)   Nap(+1)
_____ Sore (0-3)   Msg(+1)
_____ Sick (0-3)   Rest(+1)
_____ Injured (0-3)   Ice(+1)
_____ Recovery Factor   Bwork(+1)

THURSDAY   DATE

_____ Hydration (0-3) +_____ Roll(+1)
_____ Nutrition (0-3) +_____ Mwod(+1)
_____ Sleep (hrs)   +_____ Stretch(+1)
_____ Stress (0-3)   Yoga(+1)
_____ Tired(0-3)   Nap(+1)
_____ Sore (0-3)   Msg(+1)
_____ Sick (0-3)   Rest(+1)
_____ Injured (0-3)   Ice(+1)
_____ Recovery Factor   Bwork(+1)

WEEKLY LOG

FRIDAY   DATE

_____

Hydration (0-3) +_____	Roll(+1)
Nutrition (0-3) +_____	Mwod(+1)
Sleep (hrs) +_____	Stretch(+1)
Stress (0-3)	Yoga(+1)
Tired(0-3)	Nap(+1)
Sore (0-3)	Msg(+1)
Sick (0-3)	Rest(+1)
Injured (0-3)	Ice(+1)
Recovery Factor	Bwork(+1)

SATURDAY   DATE

_____

Hydration (0-3) +_____	Roll(+1)
Nutrition (0-3) +_____	Mwod(+1)
Sleep (hrs) +_____	Stretch(+1)
Stress (0-3)	Yoga(+1)
Tired(0-3)	Nap(+1)
Sore (0-3)	Msg(+1)
Sick (0-3)	Rest(+1)
Injured (0-3)	Ice(+1)
Recovery Factor	Bwork(+1)

SUNDAY   DATE

_____

Hydration (0-3) +_____	Roll(+1)
Nutrition (0-3) +_____	Mwod(+1)
Sleep (hrs) +_____	Stretch(+1)
Stress (0-3)	Yoga(+1)
Tired(0-3)	Nap(+1)
Sore (0-3)	Msg(+1)
Sick (0-3)	Rest(+1)
Injured (0-3)	Ice(+1)
Recovery Factor	Bwork(+1)

NOTES

Weekly RF Tracking

M _____
T _____
W _____
T _____
F _____
S _____
S _____
Average
Recovery Factor _____

BLOCK _____ CYCLE _____ WEEK _____

MONDAY _____ DATE _____

Hydration (0-3) + _____	Roll(+1)
Nutrition (0-3) + _____	Mwod(+1)
Sleep (hrs) + _____	Stretch(+1)
Stress (0-3)	Yoga(+1)
Tired(0-3)	Nap(+1)
Sore (0-3)	Msg(+1)
Sick (0-3)	Rest(+1)
Injured (0-3)	Ice(+1)
Recovery Factor	Bwork(+1)

TUESDAY _____ DATE _____

Hydration (0-3) + _____	Roll(+1)
Nutrition (0-3) + _____	Mwod(+1)
Sleep (hrs) + _____	Stretch(+1)
Stress (0-3)	Yoga(+1)
Tired(0-3)	Nap(+1)
Sore (0-3)	Msg(+1)
Sick (0-3)	Rest(+1)
Injured (0-3)	Ice(+1)
Recovery Factor	Bwork(+1)

WEDNESDAY _____ DATE _____

Hydration (0-3) + _____	Roll(+1)
Nutrition (0-3) + _____	Mwod(+1)
Sleep (hrs) + _____	Stretch(+1)
Stress (0-3)	Yoga(+1)
Tired(0-3)	Nap(+1)
Sore (0-3)	Msg(+1)
Sick (0-3)	Rest(+1)
Injured (0-3)	Ice(+1)
Recovery Factor	Bwork(+1)

THURSDAY _____ DATE _____

Hydration (0-3) + _____	Roll(+1)
Nutrition (0-3) + _____	Mwod(+1)
Sleep (hrs) + _____	Stretch(+1)
Stress (0-3)	Yoga(+1)
Tired(0-3)	Nap(+1)
Sore (0-3)	Msg(+1)
Sick (0-3)	Rest(+1)
Injured (0-3)	Ice(+1)
Recovery Factor	Bwork(+1)

WEEKLY LOG

FRIDAY   DATE

_____

Hydration (0-3) +_____ Roll(+1)
Nutrition (0-3) +_____ Mwod(+1)
Sleep (hrs)   +_____ Stretch(+1)
Stress (0-3)   Yoga(+1)
Tired(0-3)   Nap(+1)
Sore (0-3)   Msg(+1)
Sick (0-3)   Rest(+1)
Injured (0-3)   Ice(+1)
Recovery Factor   Bwork(+1)

SATURDAY   DATE

_____

Hydration (0-3) +_____ Roll(+1)
Nutrition (0-3) +_____ Mwod(+1)
Sleep (hrs)   +_____ Stretch(+1)
Stress (0-3)   Yoga(+1)
Tired(0-3)   Nap(+1)
Sore (0-3)   Msg(+1)
Sick (0-3)   Rest(+1)
Injured (0-3)   Ice(+1)
Recovery Factor   Bwork(+1)

SUNDAY   DATE

_____

Hydration (0-3) +_____ Roll(+1)
Nutrition (0-3) +_____ Mwod(+1)
Sleep (hrs)   +_____ Stretch(+1)
Stress (0-3)   Yoga(+1)
Tired(0-3)   Nap(+1)
Sore (0-3)   Msg(+1)
Sick (0-3)   Rest(+1)
Injured (0-3)   Ice(+1)
Recovery Factor   Bwork(+1)

NOTES

Weekly RF Tracking

M _____
T _____
W _____
T _____
F _____
S _____
S _____
Average
Recovery Factor _____

BLOCK _____ CYCLE _____ WEEK _____

MONDAY _____ DATE _____

Hydration (0-3) +_____	Roll(+1)
Nutrition (0-3) +_____	Mwod(+1)
Sleep (hrs) +_____	Stretch(+1)
Stress (0-3)	Yoga(+1)
Tired(0-3)	Nap(+1)
Sore (0-3)	Msg(+1)
Sick (0-3)	Rest(+1)
Injured (0-3)	Ice(+1)
Recovery Factor	Bwork(+1)

TUESDAY _____ DATE _____

Hydration (0-3) +_____	Roll(+1)
Nutrition (0-3) +_____	Mwod(+1)
Sleep (hrs) +_____	Stretch(+1)
Stress (0-3)	Yoga(+1)
Tired(0-3)	Nap(+1)
Sore (0-3)	Msg(+1)
Sick (0-3)	Rest(+1)
Injured (0-3)	Ice(+1)
Recovery Factor	Bwork(+1)

WEDNESDAY _____ DATE _____

Hydration (0-3) +_____	Roll(+1)
Nutrition (0-3) +_____	Mwod(+1)
Sleep (hrs) +_____	Stretch(+1)
Stress (0-3)	Yoga(+1)
Tired(0-3)	Nap(+1)
Sore (0-3)	Msg(+1)
Sick (0-3)	Rest(+1)
Injured (0-3)	Ice(+1)
Recovery Factor	Bwork(+1)

THURSDAY _____ DATE _____

Hydration (0-3) +_____	Roll(+1)
Nutrition (0-3) +_____	Mwod(+1)
Sleep (hrs) +_____	Stretch(+1)
Stress (0-3)	Yoga(+1)
Tired(0-3)	Nap(+1)
Sore (0-3)	Msg(+1)
Sick (0-3)	Rest(+1)
Injured (0-3)	Ice(+1)
Recovery Factor	Bwork(+1)

WEEKLY LOG

FRIDAY   **DATE** _____

_____

_____

_____

_____

_____

_____

_____

_____

Hydration (0-3) +_____ Roll(+1)
Nutrition (0-3) +_____ Mwod(+1)
Sleep (hrs) +_____ Stretch(+1)
Stress (0-3) Yoga(+1)
Tired(0-3) Nap(+1)
Sore (0-3) Msg(+1)
Sick (0-3) Rest(+1)
Injured (0-3) Ice(+1)
Recovery Factor Bwork(+1)

SATURDAY   **DATE** _____

_____

_____

_____

_____

_____

_____

_____

_____

Hydration (0-3) +_____ Roll(+1)
Nutrition (0-3) +_____ Mwod(+1)
Sleep (hrs) +_____ Stretch(+1)
Stress (0-3) Yoga(+1)
Tired(0-3) Nap(+1)
Sore (0-3) Msg(+1)
Sick (0-3) Rest(+1)
Injured (0-3) Ice(+1)
Recovery Factor Bwork(+1)

SUNDAY   **DATE** _____

_____

_____

_____

_____

_____

_____

_____

_____

Hydration (0-3) +_____ Roll(+1)
Nutrition (0-3) +_____ Mwod(+1)
Sleep (hrs) +_____ Stretch(+1)
Stress (0-3) Yoga(+1)
Tired(0-3) Nap(+1)
Sore (0-3) Msg(+1)
Sick (0-3) Rest(+1)
Injured (0-3) Ice(+1)
Recovery Factor Bwork(+1)

NOTES

Weekly RF Tracking
M _____
T _____
W _____
T _____
F _____
S _____
S _____
Average
Recovery Factor _____

BLOCK _____ CYCLE _____ WEEK _____

MONDAY   DATE

_____
_____
_____
_____
_____
_____
_____
_____
_____

Hydration (0-3) +_____   Roll(+1)
Nutrition (0-3) +_____   Mwod(+1)
Sleep (hrs)   +_____   Stretch(+1)
Stress (0-3)   Yoga(+1)
Tired(0-3)   Nap(+1)
Sore (0-3)   Msg(+1)
Sick (0-3)   Rest(+1)
Injured (0-3)   Ice(+1)
Recovery Factor   Bwork(+1)

TUESDAY   DATE

_____
_____
_____
_____
_____
_____
_____
_____
_____

Hydration (0-3) +_____   Roll(+1)
Nutrition (0-3) +_____   Mwod(+1)
Sleep (hrs)   +_____   Stretch(+1)
Stress (0-3)   Yoga(+1)
Tired(0-3)   Nap(+1)
Sore (0-3)   Msg(+1)
Sick (0-3)   Rest(+1)
Injured (0-3)   Ice(+1)
Recovery Factor   Bwork(+1)

WEDNESDAY   DATE

_____
_____
_____
_____
_____
_____
_____
_____
_____

Hydration (0-3) +_____   Roll(+1)
Nutrition (0-3) +_____   Mwod(+1)
Sleep (hrs)   +_____   Stretch(+1)
Stress (0-3)   Yoga(+1)
Tired(0-3)   Nap(+1)
Sore (0-3)   Msg(+1)
Sick (0-3)   Rest(+1)
Injured (0-3)   Ice(+1)
Recovery Factor   Bwork(+1)

THURSDAY   DATE

_____
_____
_____
_____
_____
_____
_____
_____
_____

Hydration (0-3) +_____   Roll(+1)
Nutrition (0-3) +_____   Mwod(+1)
Sleep (hrs)   +_____   Stretch(+1)
Stress (0-3)   Yoga(+1)
Tired(0-3)   Nap(+1)
Sore (0-3)   Msg(+1)
Sick (0-3)   Rest(+1)
Injured (0-3)   Ice(+1)
Recovery Factor   Bwork(+1)

WEEKLY LOG

FRIDAY   DATE _____

_____

Hydration (0-3) +_____		Roll(+1)
Nutrition (0-3) +_____		Mwod(+1)
Sleep (hrs) +_____		Stretch(+1)
Stress (0-3)		Yoga(+1)
Tired(0-3)		Nap(+1)
Sore (0-3)		Msg(+1)
Sick (0-3)		Rest(+1)
Injured (0-3)		Ice(+1)
Recovery Factor		Bwork(+1)

SATURDAY   DATE _____

_____

Hydration (0-3) +_____		Roll(+1)
Nutrition (0-3) +_____		Mwod(+1)
Sleep (hrs) +_____		Stretch(+1)
Stress (0-3)		Yoga(+1)
Tired(0-3)		Nap(+1)
Sore (0-3)		Msg(+1)
Sick (0-3)		Rest(+1)
Injured (0-3)		Ice(+1)
Recovery Factor		Bwork(+1)

SUNDAY   DATE _____

_____

Hydration (0-3) +_____		Roll(+1)
Nutrition (0-3) +_____		Mwod(+1)
Sleep (hrs) +_____		Stretch(+1)
Stress (0-3)		Yoga(+1)
Tired(0-3)		Nap(+1)
Sore (0-3)		Msg(+1)
Sick (0-3)		Rest(+1)
Injured (0-3)		Ice(+1)
Recovery Factor		Bwork(+1)

NOTES

Weekly RF Tracking

M _____
T _____
W _____
T _____
F _____
S _____
S _____
Average
Recovery Factor _____

BLOCK _____ CYCLE _____ WEEK _____

MONDAY   DATE

_____

Hydration (0-3) + _____		Roll(+1)
Nutrition (0-3) + _____		Mwod(+1)
Sleep (hrs) + _____		Stretch(+1)
Stress (0-3)		Yoga(+1)
Tired(0-3)		Nap(+1)
Sore (0-3)		Msg(+1)
Sick (0-3)		Rest(+1)
Injured (0-3)		Ice(+1)
Recovery Factor		Bwork(+1)

TUESDAY   DATE

_____

Hydration (0-3) + _____		Roll(+1)
Nutrition (0-3) + _____		Mwod(+1)
Sleep (hrs) + _____		Stretch(+1)
Stress (0-3)		Yoga(+1)
Tired(0-3)		Nap(+1)
Sore (0-3)		Msg(+1)
Sick (0-3)		Rest(+1)
Injured (0-3)		Ice(+1)
Recovery Factor		Bwork(+1)

WEDNESDAY   DATE

_____

Hydration (0-3) + _____		Roll(+1)
Nutrition (0-3) + _____		Mwod(+1)
Sleep (hrs) + _____		Stretch(+1)
Stress (0-3)		Yoga(+1)
Tired(0-3)		Nap(+1)
Sore (0-3)		Msg(+1)
Sick (0-3)		Rest(+1)
Injured (0-3)		Ice(+1)
Recovery Factor		Bwork(+1)

THURSDAY   DATE

_____

Hydration (0-3) + _____		Roll(+1)
Nutrition (0-3) + _____		Mwod(+1)
Sleep (hrs) + _____		Stretch(+1)
Stress (0-3)		Yoga(+1)
Tired(0-3)		Nap(+1)
Sore (0-3)		Msg(+1)
Sick (0-3)		Rest(+1)
Injured (0-3)		Ice(+1)
Recovery Factor		Bwork(+1)

WEEKLY LOG

FRIDAY   DATE

_____
_____
_____
_____
_____
_____
_____
_____
_____

Hydration (0-3) +_____ Roll(+1)
Nutrition (0-3) +_____ Mwod(+1)
Sleep (hrs)   +_____ Stretch(+1)
Stress (0-3)   Yoga(+1)
Tired(0-3)   Nap(+1)
Sore (0-3)   Msg(+1)
Sick (0-3)   Rest(+1)
Injured (0-3)   Ice(+1)
Recovery Factor   Bwork(+1)

SATURDAY   DATE

_____
_____
_____
_____
_____
_____
_____
_____
_____

Hydration (0-3) +_____ Roll(+1)
Nutrition (0-3) +_____ Mwod(+1)
Sleep (hrs)   +_____ Stretch(+1)
Stress (0-3)   Yoga(+1)
Tired(0-3)   Nap(+1)
Sore (0-3)   Msg(+1)
Sick (0-3)   Rest(+1)
Injured (0-3)   Ice(+1)
Recovery Factor   Bwork(+1)

SUNDAY   DATE

_____
_____
_____
_____
_____
_____
_____
_____
_____

Hydration (0-3) +_____ Roll(+1)
Nutrition (0-3) +_____ Mwod(+1)
Sleep (hrs)   +_____ Stretch(+1)
Stress (0-3)   Yoga(+1)
Tired(0-3)   Nap(+1)
Sore (0-3)   Msg(+1)
Sick (0-3)   Rest(+1)
Injured (0-3)   Ice(+1)
Recovery Factor   Bwork(+1)

NOTES

Weekly RF Tracking
M _____
T _____
W _____
T _____
F _____
S _____
S _____
Average
Recovery Factor _____

BLOCK _____ CYCLE _____ WEEK _____

MONDAY   DATE

Hydration (0-3) +_____	Roll(+1)
Nutrition (0-3) +_____	Mwod(+1)
Sleep (hrs) +_____	Stretch(+1)
Stress (0-3)	Yoga(+1)
Tired(0-3)	Nap(+1)
Sore (0-3)	Msg(+1)
Sick (0-3)	Rest(+1)
Injured (0-3)	Ice(+1)
Recovery Factor	Bwork(+1)

TUESDAY   DATE

Hydration (0-3) +_____	Roll(+1)
Nutrition (0-3) +_____	Mwod(+1)
Sleep (hrs) +_____	Stretch(+1)
Stress (0-3)	Yoga(+1)
Tired(0-3)	Nap(+1)
Sore (0-3)	Msg(+1)
Sick (0-3)	Rest(+1)
Injured (0-3)	Ice(+1)
Recovery Factor	Bwork(+1)

WEDNESDAY   DATE

Hydration (0-3) +_____	Roll(+1)
Nutrition (0-3) +_____	Mwod(+1)
Sleep (hrs) +_____	Stretch(+1)
Stress (0-3)	Yoga(+1)
Tired(0-3)	Nap(+1)
Sore (0-3)	Msg(+1)
Sick (0-3)	Rest(+1)
Injured (0-3)	Ice(+1)
Recovery Factor	Bwork(+1)

THURSDAY   DATE

Hydration (0-3) +_____	Roll(+1)
Nutrition (0-3) +_____	Mwod(+1)
Sleep (hrs) +_____	Stretch(+1)
Stress (0-3)	Yoga(+1)
Tired(0-3)	Nap(+1)
Sore (0-3)	Msg(+1)
Sick (0-3)	Rest(+1)
Injured (0-3)	Ice(+1)
Recovery Factor	Bwork(+1)

WEEKLY LOG

FRIDAY   DATE _____

_____

_____

_____

_____

_____

_____

_____

_____

_____

Hydration (0-3) + _____	Roll(+1)
Nutrition (0-3) + _____	Mwod(+1)
Sleep (hrs) + _____	Stretch(+1)
Stress (0-3)	Yoga(+1)
Tired(0-3)	Nap(+1)
Sore (0-3)	Msg(+1)
Sick (0-3)	Rest(+1)
Injured (0-3)	Ice(+1)
Recovery Factor	Bwork(+1)

SATURDAY   DATE _____

_____

_____

_____

_____

_____

_____

_____

_____

_____

Hydration (0-3) + _____	Roll(+1)
Nutrition (0-3) + _____	Mwod(+1)
Sleep (hrs) + _____	Stretch(+1)
Stress (0-3)	Yoga(+1)
Tired(0-3)	Nap(+1)
Sore (0-3)	Msg(+1)
Sick (0-3)	Rest(+1)
Injured (0-3)	Ice(+1)
Recovery Factor	Bwork(+1)

SUNDAY   DATE _____

_____

_____

_____

_____

_____

_____

_____

_____

_____

Hydration (0-3) + _____	Roll(+1)
Nutrition (0-3) + _____	Mwod(+1)
Sleep (hrs) + _____	Stretch(+1)
Stress (0-3)	Yoga(+1)
Tired(0-3)	Nap(+1)
Sore (0-3)	Msg(+1)
Sick (0-3)	Rest(+1)
Injured (0-3)	Ice(+1)
Recovery Factor	Bwork(+1)

NOTES

Weekly RF Tracking

M _____

T _____

W _____

T _____

F _____

S _____

S _____

Average
Recovery Factor _____

BLOCK _____ CYCLE _____ WEEK _____

MONDAY   DATE

_____
_____
_____
_____
_____
_____
_____
_____
_____

Hydration (0-3) +_____	Roll(+1)
Nutrition (0-3) +_____	Mwod(+1)
Sleep (hrs) +_____	Stretch(+1)
Stress (0-3)	Yoga(+1)
Tired(0-3)	Nap(+1)
Sore (0-3)	Msg(+1)
Sick (0-3)	Rest(+1)
Injured (0-3)	Ice(+1)
Recovery Factor	Bwork(+1)

TUESDAY   DATE

_____
_____
_____
_____
_____
_____
_____
_____
_____

Hydration (0-3) +_____	Roll(+1)
Nutrition (0-3) +_____	Mwod(+1)
Sleep (hrs) +_____	Stretch(+1)
Stress (0-3)	Yoga(+1)
Tired(0-3)	Nap(+1)
Sore (0-3)	Msg(+1)
Sick (0-3)	Rest(+1)
Injured (0-3)	Ice(+1)
Recovery Factor	Bwork(+1)

WEDNESDAY   DATE

_____
_____
_____
_____
_____
_____
_____
_____
_____

Hydration (0-3) +_____	Roll(+1)
Nutrition (0-3) +_____	Mwod(+1)
Sleep (hrs) +_____	Stretch(+1)
Stress (0-3)	Yoga(+1)
Tired(0-3)	Nap(+1)
Sore (0-3)	Msg(+1)
Sick (0-3)	Rest(+1)
Injured (0-3)	Ice(+1)
Recovery Factor	Bwork(+1)

THURSDAY   DATE

_____
_____
_____
_____
_____
_____
_____
_____
_____

Hydration (0-3) +_____	Roll(+1)
Nutrition (0-3) +_____	Mwod(+1)
Sleep (hrs) +_____	Stretch(+1)
Stress (0-3)	Yoga(+1)
Tired(0-3)	Nap(+1)
Sore (0-3)	Msg(+1)
Sick (0-3)	Rest(+1)
Injured (0-3)	Ice(+1)
Recovery Factor	Bwork(+1)

WEEKLY LOG

FRIDAY   **DATE** _____

_____

Hydration (0-3) +_____ Roll(+1)
Nutrition (0-3) +_____ Mwod(+1)
Sleep (hrs) +_____ Stretch(+1)
Stress (0-3) Yoga(+1)
Tired(0-3) Nap(+1)
Sore (0-3) Msg(+1)
Sick (0-3) Rest(+1)
Injured (0-3) Ice(+1)
Recovery Factor Bwork(+1)

SATURDAY   **DATE** _____

_____

Hydration (0-3) +_____ Roll(+1)
Nutrition (0-3) +_____ Mwod(+1)
Sleep (hrs) +_____ Stretch(+1)
Stress (0-3) Yoga(+1)
Tired(0-3) Nap(+1)
Sore (0-3) Msg(+1)
Sick (0-3) Rest(+1)
Injured (0-3) Ice(+1)
Recovery Factor Bwork(+1)

SUNDAY   **DATE** _____

_____

Hydration (0-3) +_____ Roll(+1)
Nutrition (0-3) +_____ Mwod(+1)
Sleep (hrs) +_____ Stretch(+1)
Stress (0-3) Yoga(+1)
Tired(0-3) Nap(+1)
Sore (0-3) Msg(+1)
Sick (0-3) Rest(+1)
Injured (0-3) Ice(+1)
Recovery Factor Bwork(+1)

NOTES

Weekly RF Tracking
M _____
T _____
W _____
T _____
F _____
S _____
S _____
Average
Recovery Factor _____

BLOCK _____ CYCLE _____ WEEK _____

MONDAY   DATE _____

_____

Hydration (0-3) + _____		Roll(+1)
Nutrition (0-3) + _____		Mwod(+1)
Sleep (hrs) + _____		Stretch(+1)
Stress (0-3)		Yoga(+1)
Tired(0-3)		Nap(+1)
Sore (0-3)		Msg(+1)
Sick (0-3)		Rest(+1)
Injured (0-3)		Ice(+1)
Recovery Factor		Bwork(+1)

TUESDAY   DATE _____

_____

Hydration (0-3) + _____		Roll(+1)
Nutrition (0-3) + _____		Mwod(+1)
Sleep (hrs) + _____		Stretch(+1)
Stress (0-3)		Yoga(+1)
Tired(0-3)		Nap(+1)
Sore (0-3)		Msg(+1)
Sick (0-3)		Rest(+1)
Injured (0-3)		Ice(+1)
Recovery Factor		Bwork(+1)

WEDNESDAY   DATE _____

_____

Hydration (0-3) + _____		Roll(+1)
Nutrition (0-3) + _____		Mwod(+1)
Sleep (hrs) + _____		Stretch(+1)
Stress (0-3)		Yoga(+1)
Tired(0-3)		Nap(+1)
Sore (0-3)		Msg(+1)
Sick (0-3)		Rest(+1)
Injured (0-3)		Ice(+1)
Recovery Factor		Bwork(+1)

THURSDAY   DATE _____

_____

Hydration (0-3) + _____		Roll(+1)
Nutrition (0-3) + _____		Mwod(+1)
Sleep (hrs) + _____		Stretch(+1)
Stress (0-3)		Yoga(+1)
Tired(0-3)		Nap(+1)
Sore (0-3)		Msg(+1)
Sick (0-3)		Rest(+1)
Injured (0-3)		Ice(+1)
Recovery Factor		Bwork(+1)

WEEKLY LOG

FRIDAY   DATE

_____

Hydration (0-3) +_____	Roll(+1)
Nutrition (0-3) +_____	Mwod(+1)
Sleep (hrs) +_____	Stretch(+1)
Stress (0-3)	Yoga(+1)
Tired(0-3)	Nap(+1)
Sore (0-3)	Msg(+1)
Sick (0-3)	Rest(+1)
Injured (0-3)	Ice(+1)
Recovery Factor	Bwork(+1)

SATURDAY   DATE

_____

Hydration (0-3) +_____	Roll(+1)
Nutrition (0-3) +_____	Mwod(+1)
Sleep (hrs) +_____	Stretch(+1)
Stress (0-3)	Yoga(+1)
Tired(0-3)	Nap(+1)
Sore (0-3)	Msg(+1)
Sick (0-3)	Rest(+1)
Injured (0-3)	Ice(+1)
Recovery Factor	Bwork(+1)

SUNDAY   DATE

_____

Hydration (0-3) +_____	Roll(+1)
Nutrition (0-3) +_____	Mwod(+1)
Sleep (hrs) +_____	Stretch(+1)
Stress (0-3)	Yoga(+1)
Tired(0-3)	Nap(+1)
Sore (0-3)	Msg(+1)
Sick (0-3)	Rest(+1)
Injured (0-3)	Ice(+1)
Recovery Factor	Bwork(+1)

NOTES

Weekly RF Tracking

M _____
T _____
W _____
T _____
F _____
S _____
S _____
Average
Recovery Factor _____

BLOCK _____ CYCLE _____ WEEK _____

MONDAY   DATE _____

Hydration (0-3) +_____	Roll(+1)
Nutrition (0-3) +_____	Mwod(+1)
Sleep (hrs) +_____	Stretch(+1)
Stress (0-3)	Yoga(+1)
Tired(0-3)	Nap(+1)
Sore (0-3)	Msg(+1)
Sick (0-3)	Rest(+1)
Injured (0-3)	Ice(+1)
Recovery Factor	Bwork(+1)

TUESDAY   DATE _____

Hydration (0-3) +_____	Roll(+1)
Nutrition (0-3) +_____	Mwod(+1)
Sleep (hrs) +_____	Stretch(+1)
Stress (0-3)	Yoga(+1)
Tired(0-3)	Nap(+1)
Sore (0-3)	Msg(+1)
Sick (0-3)	Rest(+1)
Injured (0-3)	Ice(+1)
Recovery Factor	Bwork(+1)

WEDNESDAY   DATE _____

Hydration (0-3) +_____	Roll(+1)
Nutrition (0-3) +_____	Mwod(+1)
Sleep (hrs) +_____	Stretch(+1)
Stress (0-3)	Yoga(+1)
Tired(0-3)	Nap(+1)
Sore (0-3)	Msg(+1)
Sick (0-3)	Rest(+1)
Injured (0-3)	Ice(+1)
Recovery Factor	Bwork(+1)

THURSDAY   DATE _____

Hydration (0-3) +_____	Roll(+1)
Nutrition (0-3) +_____	Mwod(+1)
Sleep (hrs) +_____	Stretch(+1)
Stress (0-3)	Yoga(+1)
Tired(0-3)	Nap(+1)
Sore (0-3)	Msg(+1)
Sick (0-3)	Rest(+1)
Injured (0-3)	Ice(+1)
Recovery Factor	Bwork(+1)

WEEKLY LOG

FRIDAY   DATE _____

_____

_____

_____

_____

_____

_____

_____

_____

Hydration (0-3) +_____	Roll(+1)
Nutrition (0-3) +_____	Mwod(+1)
Sleep (hrs) +_____	Stretch(+1)
Stress (0-3)	Yoga(+1)
Tired(0-3)	Nap(+1)
Sore (0-3)	Msg(+1)
Sick (0-3)	Rest(+1)
Injured (0-3)	Ice(+1)
Recovery Factor	Bwork(+1)

SATURDAY   DATE _____

_____

_____

_____

_____

_____

_____

_____

_____

Hydration (0-3) +_____	Roll(+1)
Nutrition (0-3) +_____	Mwod(+1)
Sleep (hrs) +_____	Stretch(+1)
Stress (0-3)	Yoga(+1)
Tired(0-3)	Nap(+1)
Sore (0-3)	Msg(+1)
Sick (0-3)	Rest(+1)
Injured (0-3)	Ice(+1)
Recovery Factor	Bwork(+1)

SUNDAY   DATE _____

_____

_____

_____

_____

_____

_____

_____

_____

Hydration (0-3) +_____	Roll(+1)
Nutrition (0-3) +_____	Mwod(+1)
Sleep (hrs) +_____	Stretch(+1)
Stress (0-3)	Yoga(+1)
Tired(0-3)	Nap(+1)
Sore (0-3)	Msg(+1)
Sick (0-3)	Rest(+1)
Injured (0-3)	Ice(+1)
Recovery Factor	Bwork(+1)

NOTES

Weekly RF Tracking

M _____

T _____

W _____

T _____

F _____

S _____

S _____

Average
Recovery Factor _____

BLOCK _____ CYCLE _____ WEEK _____

MONDAY   DATE

Hydration (0-3) + _____	Roll(+1)
Nutrition (0-3) + _____	Mwod(+1)
Sleep (hrs) + _____	Stretch(+1)
Stress (0-3)	Yoga(+1)
Tired(0-3)	Nap(+1)
Sore (0-3)	Msg(+1)
Sick (0-3)	Rest(+1)
Injured (0-3)	Ice(+1)
Recovery Factor	Bwork(+1)

TUESDAY   DATE

Hydration (0-3) + _____	Roll(+1)
Nutrition (0-3) + _____	Mwod(+1)
Sleep (hrs) + _____	Stretch(+1)
Stress (0-3)	Yoga(+1)
Tired(0-3)	Nap(+1)
Sore (0-3)	Msg(+1)
Sick (0-3)	Rest(+1)
Injured (0-3)	Ice(+1)
Recovery Factor	Bwork(+1)

WEDNESDAY   DATE

Hydration (0-3) + _____	Roll(+1)
Nutrition (0-3) + _____	Mwod(+1)
Sleep (hrs) + _____	Stretch(+1)
Stress (0-3)	Yoga(+1)
Tired(0-3)	Nap(+1)
Sore (0-3)	Msg(+1)
Sick (0-3)	Rest(+1)
Injured (0-3)	Ice(+1)
Recovery Factor	Bwork(+1)

THURSDAY   DATE

Hydration (0-3) + _____	Roll(+1)
Nutrition (0-3) + _____	Mwod(+1)
Sleep (hrs) + _____	Stretch(+1)
Stress (0-3)	Yoga(+1)
Tired(0-3)	Nap(+1)
Sore (0-3)	Msg(+1)
Sick (0-3)	Rest(+1)
Injured (0-3)	Ice(+1)
Recovery Factor	Bwork(+1)

WEEKLY LOG

FRIDAY   DATE

_____
_____
_____
_____
_____
_____
_____
_____
_____

Hydration (0-3) +_____ Roll(+1)
Nutrition (0-3) +_____ Mwod(+1)
Sleep (hrs)   +_____ Stretch(+1)
Stress (0-3)   Yoga(+1)
Tired(0-3)   Nap(+1)
Sore (0-3)   Msg(+1)
Sick (0-3)   Rest(+1)
Injured (0-3)   Ice(+1)
Recovery Factor   Bwork(+1)

SATURDAY   DATE

_____
_____
_____
_____
_____
_____
_____
_____
_____

Hydration (0-3) +_____ Roll(+1)
Nutrition (0-3) +_____ Mwod(+1)
Sleep (hrs)   +_____ Stretch(+1)
Stress (0-3)   Yoga(+1)
Tired(0-3)   Nap(+1)
Sore (0-3)   Msg(+1)
Sick (0-3)   Rest(+1)
Injured (0-3)   Ice(+1)
Recovery Factor   Bwork(+1)

SUNDAY   DATE

_____
_____
_____
_____
_____
_____
_____
_____
_____

Hydration (0-3) +_____ Roll(+1)
Nutrition (0-3) +_____ Mwod(+1)
Sleep (hrs)   +_____ Stretch(+1)
Stress (0-3)   Yoga(+1)
Tired(0-3)   Nap(+1)
Sore (0-3)   Msg(+1)
Sick (0-3)   Rest(+1)
Injured (0-3)   Ice(+1)
Recovery Factor   Bwork(+1)

NOTES

Weekly RF Tracking

M _____
T _____
W _____
T _____
F _____
S _____
S _____
Average
Recovery Factor _____

BLOCK _____ CYCLE _____ WEEK _____

MONDAY   DATE

Hydration (0-3) + _____	Roll(+1)
Nutrition (0-3) + _____	Mwod(+1)
Sleep (hrs) + _____	Stretch(+1)
Stress (0-3)	Yoga(+1)
Tired(0-3)	Nap(+1)
Sore (0-3)	Msg(+1)
Sick (0-3)	Rest(+1)
Injured (0-3)	Ice(+1)
Recovery Factor	Bwork(+1)

TUESDAY   DATE

Hydration (0-3) + _____	Roll(+1)
Nutrition (0-3) + _____	Mwod(+1)
Sleep (hrs) + _____	Stretch(+1)
Stress (0-3)	Yoga(+1)
Tired(0-3)	Nap(+1)
Sore (0-3)	Msg(+1)
Sick (0-3)	Rest(+1)
Injured (0-3)	Ice(+1)
Recovery Factor	Bwork(+1)

WEDNESDAY   DATE

Hydration (0-3) + _____	Roll(+1)
Nutrition (0-3) + _____	Mwod(+1)
Sleep (hrs) + _____	Stretch(+1)
Stress (0-3)	Yoga(+1)
Tired(0-3)	Nap(+1)
Sore (0-3)	Msg(+1)
Sick (0-3)	Rest(+1)
Injured (0-3)	Ice(+1)
Recovery Factor	Bwork(+1)

THURSDAY   DATE

Hydration (0-3) + _____	Roll(+1)
Nutrition (0-3) + _____	Mwod(+1)
Sleep (hrs) + _____	Stretch(+1)
Stress (0-3)	Yoga(+1)
Tired(0-3)	Nap(+1)
Sore (0-3)	Msg(+1)
Sick (0-3)	Rest(+1)
Injured (0-3)	Ice(+1)
Recovery Factor	Bwork(+1)

WEEKLY LOG

FRIDAY   DATE _____

_____   Hydration (0-3) +_____ Roll(+1)
_____   Nutrition (0-3) +_____ Mwod(+1)
_____   Sleep (hrs)   +_____ Stretch(+1)
_____   Stress (0-3)   Yoga(+1)
_____   Tired(0-3)   Nap(+1)
_____   Sore (0-3)   Msg(+1)
_____   Sick (0-3)   Rest(+1)
_____   Injured (0-3)   Ice(+1)
_____   Recovery Factor   Bwork(+1)

SATURDAY   DATE _____

_____   Hydration (0-3) +_____ Roll(+1)
_____   Nutrition (0-3) +_____ Mwod(+1)
_____   Sleep (hrs)   +_____ Stretch(+1)
_____   Stress (0-3)   Yoga(+1)
_____   Tired(0-3)   Nap(+1)
_____   Sore (0-3)   Msg(+1)
_____   Sick (0-3)   Rest(+1)
_____   Injured (0-3)   Ice(+1)
_____   Recovery Factor   Bwork(+1)

SUNDAY   DATE _____

_____   Hydration (0-3) +_____ Roll(+1)
_____   Nutrition (0-3) +_____ Mwod(+1)
_____   Sleep (hrs)   +_____ Stretch(+1)
_____   Stress (0-3)   Yoga(+1)
_____   Tired(0-3)   Nap(+1)
_____   Sore (0-3)   Msg(+1)
_____   Sick (0-3)   Rest(+1)
_____   Injured (0-3)   Ice(+1)
_____   Recovery Factor   Bwork(+1)

N O T E S

Weekly RF Tracking

M _____
T _____
W _____
T _____
F _____
S _____
S _____
Average
Recovery Factor _____

BLOCK _____ CYCLE _____ WEEK _____

MONDAY   DATE

_____

Hydration (0-3) + _____		Roll(+1)
Nutrition (0-3) + _____		Mwod(+1)
Sleep (hrs) + _____		Stretch(+1)
Stress (0-3)		Yoga(+1)
Tired(0-3)		Nap(+1)
Sore (0-3)		Msg(+1)
Sick (0-3)		Rest(+1)
Injured (0-3)		Ice(+1)
Recovery Factor		Bwork(+1)

TUESDAY   DATE

_____

Hydration (0-3) + _____		Roll(+1)
Nutrition (0-3) + _____		Mwod(+1)
Sleep (hrs) + _____		Stretch(+1)
Stress (0-3)		Yoga(+1)
Tired(0-3)		Nap(+1)
Sore (0-3)		Msg(+1)
Sick (0-3)		Rest(+1)
Injured (0-3)		Ice(+1)
Recovery Factor		Bwork(+1)

WEDNESDAY   DATE

_____

Hydration (0-3) + _____		Roll(+1)
Nutrition (0-3) + _____		Mwod(+1)
Sleep (hrs) + _____		Stretch(+1)
Stress (0-3)		Yoga(+1)
Tired(0-3)		Nap(+1)
Sore (0-3)		Msg(+1)
Sick (0-3)		Rest(+1)
Injured (0-3)		Ice(+1)
Recovery Factor		Bwork(+1)

THURSDAY   DATE

_____

Hydration (0-3) + _____		Roll(+1)
Nutrition (0-3) + _____		Mwod(+1)
Sleep (hrs) + _____		Stretch(+1)
Stress (0-3)		Yoga(+1)
Tired(0-3)		Nap(+1)
Sore (0-3)		Msg(+1)
Sick (0-3)		Rest(+1)
Injured (0-3)		Ice(+1)
Recovery Factor		Bwork(+1)

WEEKLY LOG

FRIDAY   DATE _____

_____

_____

_____

_____

_____

_____

_____

_____

_____

Hydration (0-3)	+ _____	Roll(+1)
Nutrition (0-3)	+ _____	Mwod(+1)
Sleep (hrs)	+ _____	Stretch(+1)
Stress (0-3)	-	Yoga(+1)
Tired(0-3)	-	Nap(+1)
Sore (0-3)	-	Msg(+1)
Sick (0-3)	-	Rest(+1)
Injured (0-3)	-	Ice(+1)
Recovery Factor		Bwork(+1)

SATURDAY   DATE _____

_____

_____

_____

_____

_____

_____

_____

_____

_____

Hydration (0-3)	+ _____	Roll(+1)
Nutrition (0-3)	+ _____	Mwod(+1)
Sleep (hrs)	+ _____	Stretch(+1)
Stress (0-3)	-	Yoga(+1)
Tired(0-3)	-	Nap(+1)
Sore (0-3)	-	Msg(+1)
Sick (0-3)	-	Rest(+1)
Injured (0-3)	-	Ice(+1)
Recovery Factor		Bwork(+1)

SUNDAY   DATE _____

_____

_____

_____

_____

_____

_____

_____

_____

_____

Hydration (0-3)	+ _____	Roll(+1)
Nutrition (0-3)	+ _____	Mwod(+1)
Sleep (hrs)	+ _____	Stretch(+1)
Stress (0-3)	-	Yoga(+1)
Tired(0-3)	-	Nap(+1)
Sore (0-3)	-	Msg(+1)
Sick (0-3)	-	Rest(+1)
Injured (0-3)	-	Ice(+1)
Recovery Factor		Bwork(+1)

NOTES

Weekly RF Tracking

M _____

T _____

W _____

T _____

F _____

S _____

S _____

Average
Recovery Factor _____

BLOCK _____ CYCLE _____ WEEK _____

MONDAY   DATE _____

Hydration (0-3) +_____	Roll(+1)
Nutrition (0-3) +_____	Mwod(+1)
Sleep (hrs) +_____	Stretch(+1)
Stress (0-3)	Yoga(+1)
Tired(0-3)	Nap(+1)
Sore (0-3)	Msg(+1)
Sick (0-3)	Rest(+1)
Injured (0-3)	Ice(+1)
Recovery Factor	Bwork(+1)

TUESDAY   DATE _____

Hydration (0-3) +_____	Roll(+1)
Nutrition (0-3) +_____	Mwod(+1)
Sleep (hrs) +_____	Stretch(+1)
Stress (0-3)	Yoga(+1)
Tired(0-3)	Nap(+1)
Sore (0-3)	Msg(+1)
Sick (0-3)	Rest(+1)
Injured (0-3)	Ice(+1)
Recovery Factor	Bwork(+1)

WEDNESDAY   DATE _____

Hydration (0-3) +_____	Roll(+1)
Nutrition (0-3) +_____	Mwod(+1)
Sleep (hrs) +_____	Stretch(+1)
Stress (0-3)	Yoga(+1)
Tired(0-3)	Nap(+1)
Sore (0-3)	Msg(+1)
Sick (0-3)	Rest(+1)
Injured (0-3)	Ice(+1)
Recovery Factor	Bwork(+1)

THURSDAY   DATE _____

Hydration (0-3) +_____	Roll(+1)
Nutrition (0-3) +_____	Mwod(+1)
Sleep (hrs) +_____	Stretch(+1)
Stress (0-3)	Yoga(+1)
Tired(0-3)	Nap(+1)
Sore (0-3)	Msg(+1)
Sick (0-3)	Rest(+1)
Injured (0-3)	Ice(+1)
Recovery Factor	Bwork(+1)

WEEKLY LOG

FRIDAY   **DATE**

_____

_____   Hydration (0-3) +_____ Roll(+1)

_____   Nutrition (0-3) +_____ Mwod(+1)

_____   Sleep (hrs)   +_____ Stretch(+1)

_____   Stress (0-3)   Yoga(+1)

_____   Tired(0-3)   Nap(+1)

   Sore (0-3)   Msg(+1)

   Sick (0-3)   Rest(+1)

_____   Injured (0-3)   Ice(+1)

_____   Recovery Factor   Bwork(+1)

SATURDAY   **DATE**

_____   Hydration (0-3) +_____ Roll(+1)

_____   Nutrition (0-3) +_____ Mwod(+1)

_____   Sleep (hrs)   +_____ Stretch(+1)

_____   Stress (0-3)   Yoga(+1)

_____   Tired(0-3)   Nap(+1)

   Sore (0-3)   Msg(+1)

   Sick (0-3)   Rest(+1)

_____   Injured (0-3)   Ice(+1)

_____   Recovery Factor   Bwork(+1)

SUNDAY   **DATE**

_____   Hydration (0-3) +_____ Roll(+1)

_____   Nutrition (0-3) +_____ Mwod(+1)

_____   Sleep (hrs)   +_____ Stretch(+1)

_____   Stress (0-3)   Yoga(+1)

_____   Tired(0-3)   Nap(+1)

   Sore (0-3)   Msg(+1)

   Sick (0-3)   Rest(+1)

_____   Injured (0-3)   Ice(+1)

_____   Recovery Factor   Bwork(+1)

NOTES

Weekly RF Tracking

M _____

T _____

W _____

T _____

F _____

S _____

S _____

Average
Recovery Factor _____

BLOCK _____ CYCLE _____ WEEK _____

MONDAY   DATE _____

_____	Hydration (0-3) + _____ Roll(+1)
_____	Nutrition (0-3) + _____ Mwod(+1)
_____	Sleep (hrs) + _____ Stretch(+1)
_____	Stress (0-3) Yoga(+1)
_____	Tired(0-3) Nap(+1)
_____	Sore (0-3) Msg(+1)
_____	Sick (0-3) Rest(+1)
_____	Injured (0-3) Ice(+1)
_____	Recovery Factor Bwork(+1)

TUESDAY   DATE _____

_____	Hydration (0-3) + _____ Roll(+1)
_____	Nutrition (0-3) + _____ Mwod(+1)
_____	Sleep (hrs) + _____ Stretch(+1)
_____	Stress (0-3) Yoga(+1)
_____	Tired(0-3) Nap(+1)
_____	Sore (0-3) Msg(+1)
_____	Sick (0-3) Rest(+1)
_____	Injured (0-3) Ice(+1)
_____	Recovery Factor Bwork(+1)

WEDNESDAY   DATE _____

_____	Hydration (0-3) + _____ Roll(+1)
_____	Nutrition (0-3) + _____ Mwod(+1)
_____	Sleep (hrs) + _____ Stretch(+1)
_____	Stress (0-3) Yoga(+1)
_____	Tired(0-3) Nap(+1)
_____	Sore (0-3) Msg(+1)
_____	Sick (0-3) Rest(+1)
_____	Injured (0-3) Ice(+1)
_____	Recovery Factor Bwork(+1)

THURSDAY   DATE _____

_____	Hydration (0-3) + _____ Roll(+1)
_____	Nutrition (0-3) + _____ Mwod(+1)
_____	Sleep (hrs) + _____ Stretch(+1)
_____	Stress (0-3) Yoga(+1)
_____	Tired(0-3) Nap(+1)
_____	Sore (0-3) Msg(+1)
_____	Sick (0-3) Rest(+1)
_____	Injured (0-3) Ice(+1)
_____	Recovery Factor Bwork(+1)

WEEKLY LOG

FRIDAY　　　**DATE** _____

_____

_____

_____

_____

_____

_____

_____

_____

Hydration (0-3)	+_____	Roll(+1)
Nutrition (0-3)	+_____	Mwod(+1)
Sleep (hrs)	+_____	Stretch(+1)
Stress (0-3)		Yoga(+1)
Tired(0-3)		Nap(+1)
Sore (0-3)		Msg(+1)
Sick (0-3)		Rest(+1)
Injured (0-3)		Ice(+1)
Recovery Factor		Bwork(+1)

SATURDAY　　　**DATE** _____

_____

_____

_____

_____

_____

_____

_____

_____

Hydration (0-3)	+_____	Roll(+1)
Nutrition (0-3)	+_____	Mwod(+1)
Sleep (hrs)	+_____	Stretch(+1)
Stress (0-3)		Yoga(+1)
Tired(0-3)		Nap(+1)
Sore (0-3)		Msg(+1)
Sick (0-3)		Rest(+1)
Injured (0-3)		Ice(+1)
Recovery Factor		Bwork(+1)

SUNDAY　　　**DATE** _____

_____

_____

_____

_____

_____

_____

_____

_____

Hydration (0-3)	+_____	Roll(+1)
Nutrition (0-3)	+_____	Mwod(+1)
Sleep (hrs)	+_____	Stretch(+1)
Stress (0-3)		Yoga(+1)
Tired(0-3)		Nap(+1)
Sore (0-3)		Msg(+1)
Sick (0-3)		Rest(+1)
Injured (0-3)		Ice(+1)
Recovery Factor		Bwork(+1)

NOTES

Weekly RF Tracking

M _____

T _____

W _____

T _____

F _____

S _____

S _____

Average
Recovery Factor _____

BLOCK _____ CYCLE _____ WEEK _____

MONDAY DATE

_____
_____
_____
_____
_____
_____
_____
_____
_____

Hydration (0-3) +_____		Roll(+1)
Nutrition (0-3) +_____		Mwod(+1)
Sleep (hrs) +_____		Stretch(+1)
Stress (0-3)		Yoga(+1)
Tired(0-3)		Nap(+1)
Sore (0-3)		Msg(+1)
Sick (0-3)		Rest(+1)
Injured (0-3)		Ice(+1)
Recovery Factor		Bwork(+1)

TUESDAY DATE

_____
_____
_____
_____
_____
_____
_____
_____

Hydration (0-3) +_____		Roll(+1)
Nutrition (0-3) +_____		Mwod(+1)
Sleep (hrs) +_____		Stretch(+1)
Stress (0-3)		Yoga(+1)
Tired(0-3)		Nap(+1)
Sore (0-3)		Msg(+1)
Sick (0-3)		Rest(+1)
Injured (0-3)		Ice(+1)
Recovery Factor		Bwork(+1)

WEDNESDAY DATE

_____
_____
_____
_____
_____
_____
_____
_____

Hydration (0-3) +_____		Roll(+1)
Nutrition (0-3) +_____		Mwod(+1)
Sleep (hrs) +_____		Stretch(+1)
Stress (0-3)		Yoga(+1)
Tired(0-3)		Nap(+1)
Sore (0-3)		Msg(+1)
Sick (0-3)		Rest(+1)
Injured (0-3)		Ice(+1)
Recovery Factor		Bwork(+1)

THURSDAY DATE

_____
_____
_____
_____
_____
_____
_____
_____
_____

Hydration (0-3) +_____		Roll(+1)
Nutrition (0-3) +_____		Mwod(+1)
Sleep (hrs) +_____		Stretch(+1)
Stress (0-3)		Yoga(+1)
Tired(0-3)		Nap(+1)
Sore (0-3)		Msg(+1)
Sick (0-3)		Rest(+1)
Injured (0-3)		Ice(+1)
Recovery Factor		Bwork(+1)

WEEKLY LOG

FRIDAY   **DATE**

Hydration (0-3) + _____	Roll(+1)
Nutrition (0-3) + _____	Mwod(+1)
Sleep (hrs) + _____	Stretch(+1)
Stress (0-3)	Yoga(+1)
Tired(0-3)	Nap(+1)
Sore (0-3)	Msg(+1)
Sick (0-3)	Rest(+1)
Injured (0-3)	Ice(+1)
Recovery Factor	Bwork(+1)

SATURDAY   **DATE**

Hydration (0-3) + _____	Roll(+1)
Nutrition (0-3) + _____	Mwod(+1)
Sleep (hrs) + _____	Stretch(+1)
Stress (0-3)	Yoga(+1)
Tired(0-3)	Nap(+1)
Sore (0-3)	Msg(+1)
Sick (0-3)	Rest(+1)
Injured (0-3)	Ice(+1)
Recovery Factor	Bwork(+1)

SUNDAY   **DATE**

Hydration (0-3) + _____	Roll(+1)
Nutrition (0-3) + _____	Mwod(+1)
Sleep (hrs) + _____	Stretch(+1)
Stress (0-3)	Yoga(+1)
Tired(0-3)	Nap(+1)
Sore (0-3)	Msg(+1)
Sick (0-3)	Rest(+1)
Injured (0-3)	Ice(+1)
Recovery Factor	Bwork(+1)

NOTES

Weekly RF Tracking

M _____
T _____
W _____
T _____
F _____
S _____
S _____
Average
Recovery Factor _____

BLOCK _____ CYCLE _____ WEEK _____

MONDAY   DATE _____

_____

Hydration (0-3) +_____	Roll(+1)
Nutrition (0-3) +_____	Mwod(+1)
Sleep (hrs) +_____	Stretch(+1)
Stress (0-3)	Yoga(+1)
Tired(0-3)	Nap(+1)
Sore (0-3)	Msg(+1)
Sick (0-3)	Rest(+1)
Injured (0-3)	Ice(+1)
Recovery Factor	Bwork(+1)

TUESDAY   DATE _____

_____

Hydration (0-3) +_____	Roll(+1)
Nutrition (0-3) +_____	Mwod(+1)
Sleep (hrs) +_____	Stretch(+1)
Stress (0-3)	Yoga(+1)
Tired(0-3)	Nap(+1)
Sore (0-3)	Msg(+1)
Sick (0-3)	Rest(+1)
Injured (0-3)	Ice(+1)
Recovery Factor	Bwork(+1)

WEDNESDAY   DATE _____

_____

Hydration (0-3) +_____	Roll(+1)
Nutrition (0-3) +_____	Mwod(+1)
Sleep (hrs) +_____	Stretch(+1)
Stress (0-3)	Yoga(+1)
Tired(0-3)	Nap(+1)
Sore (0-3)	Msg(+1)
Sick (0-3)	Rest(+1)
Injured (0-3)	Ice(+1)
Recovery Factor	Bwork(+1)

THURSDAY   DATE _____

_____

Hydration (0-3) +_____	Roll(+1)
Nutrition (0-3) +_____	Mwod(+1)
Sleep (hrs) +_____	Stretch(+1)
Stress (0-3)	Yoga(+1)
Tired(0-3)	Nap(+1)
Sore (0-3)	Msg(+1)
Sick (0-3)	Rest(+1)
Injured (0-3)	Ice(+1)
Recovery Factor	Bwork(+1)

WEEKLY LOG

FRIDAY — DATE _____

_____

Hydration (0-3) +_____ Roll(+1)
Nutrition (0-3) +_____ Mwod(+1)
Sleep (hrs) +_____ Stretch(+1)
Stress (0-3) Yoga(+1)
Tired(0-3) Nap(+1)
Sore (0-3) Msg(+1)
Sick (0-3) Rest(+1)
Injured (0-3) Ice(+1)
Recovery Factor Bwork(+1)

SATURDAY — DATE _____

_____

Hydration (0-3) +_____ Roll(+1)
Nutrition (0-3) +_____ Mwod(+1)
Sleep (hrs) +_____ Stretch(+1)
Stress (0-3) Yoga(+1)
Tired(0-3) Nap(+1)
Sore (0-3) Msg(+1)
Sick (0-3) Rest(+1)
Injured (0-3) Ice(+1)
Recovery Factor Bwork(+1)

SUNDAY — DATE _____

_____

Hydration (0-3) +_____ Roll(+1)
Nutrition (0-3) +_____ Mwod(+1)
Sleep (hrs) +_____ Stretch(+1)
Stress (0-3) Yoga(+1)
Tired(0-3) Nap(+1)
Sore (0-3) Msg(+1)
Sick (0-3) Rest(+1)
Injured (0-3) Ice(+1)
Recovery Factor Bwork(+1)

NOTES

Weekly RF Tracking
M _____
T _____
W _____
T _____
F _____
S _____
S _____
Average
Recovery Factor _____

BLOCK _____ CYCLE _____ WEEK _____

MONDAY   DATE

Hydration (0-3) +_____	Roll(+1)
Nutrition (0-3) +_____	Mwod(+1)
Sleep (hrs) +_____	Stretch(+1)
Stress (0-3)	Yoga(+1)
Tired(0-3)	Nap(+1)
Sore (0-3)	Msg(+1)
Sick (0-3)	Rest(+1)
Injured (0-3)	Ice(+1)
Recovery Factor	Bwork(+1)

TUESDAY   DATE

Hydration (0-3) +_____	Roll(+1)
Nutrition (0-3) +_____	Mwod(+1)
Sleep (hrs) +_____	Stretch(+1)
Stress (0-3)	Yoga(+1)
Tired(0-3)	Nap(+1)
Sore (0-3)	Msg(+1)
Sick (0-3)	Rest(+1)
Injured (0-3)	Ice(+1)
Recovery Factor	Bwork(+1)

WEDNESDAY   DATE

Hydration (0-3) +_____	Roll(+1)
Nutrition (0-3) +_____	Mwod(+1)
Sleep (hrs) +_____	Stretch(+1)
Stress (0-3)	Yoga(+1)
Tired(0-3)	Nap(+1)
Sore (0-3)	Msg(+1)
Sick (0-3)	Rest(+1)
Injured (0-3)	Ice(+1)
Recovery Factor	Bwork(+1)

THURSDAY   DATE

Hydration (0-3) +_____	Roll(+1)
Nutrition (0-3) +_____	Mwod(+1)
Sleep (hrs) +_____	Stretch(+1)
Stress (0-3)	Yoga(+1)
Tired(0-3)	Nap(+1)
Sore (0-3)	Msg(+1)
Sick (0-3)	Rest(+1)
Injured (0-3)	Ice(+1)
Recovery Factor	Bwork(+1)

WEEKLY LOG

FRIDAY   DATE _____

_____   Hydration (0-3) +_____ Roll(+1)
_____   Nutrition (0-3) +_____ Mwod(+1)
_____   Sleep (hrs)   +_____ Stretch(+1)
_____   Stress (0-3)   Yoga(+1)
_____   Tired(0-3)   Nap(+1)
_____   Sore (0-3)   Msg(+1)
_____   Sick (0-3)   Rest(+1)
_____   Injured (0-3)   Ice(+1)
_____   Recovery Factor   Bwork(+1)

SATURDAY   DATE _____

_____   Hydration (0-3) +_____ Roll(+1)
_____   Nutrition (0-3) +_____ Mwod(+1)
_____   Sleep (hrs)   +_____ Stretch(+1)
_____   Stress (0-3)   Yoga(+1)
_____   Tired(0-3)   Nap(+1)
_____   Sore (0-3)   Msg(+1)
_____   Sick (0-3)   Rest(+1)
_____   Injured (0-3)   Ice(+1)
_____   Recovery Factor   Bwork(+1)

SUNDAY   DATE _____

_____   Hydration (0-3) +_____ Roll(+1)
_____   Nutrition (0-3) +_____ Mwod(+1)
_____   Sleep (hrs)   +_____ Stretch(+1)
_____   Stress (0-3)   Yoga(+1)
_____   Tired(0-3)   Nap(+1)
_____   Sore (0-3)   Msg(+1)
_____   Sick (0-3)   Rest(+1)
_____   Injured (0-3)   Ice(+1)
_____   Recovery Factor   Bwork(+1)

NOTES

Weekly RF Tracking

M _____
T _____
W _____
T _____
F _____
S _____
S _____
Average
Recovery Factor _____

BLOCK _____ CYCLE _____ WEEK _____

MONDAY   DATE

Hydration (0-3) +_____	Roll(+1)
Nutrition (0-3) +_____	Mwod(+1)
Sleep (hrs) +_____	Stretch(+1)
Stress (0-3)	Yoga(+1)
Tired(0-3)	Nap(+1)
Sore (0-3)	Msg(+1)
Sick (0-3)	Rest(+1)
Injured (0-3)	Ice(+1)
Recovery Factor	Bwork(+1)

TUESDAY   DATE

Hydration (0-3) +_____	Roll(+1)
Nutrition (0-3) +_____	Mwod(+1)
Sleep (hrs) +_____	Stretch(+1)
Stress (0-3)	Yoga(+1)
Tired(0-3)	Nap(+1)
Sore (0-3)	Msg(+1)
Sick (0-3)	Rest(+1)
Injured (0-3)	Ice(+1)
Recovery Factor	Bwork(+1)

WEDNESDAY   DATE

Hydration (0-3) +_____	Roll(+1)
Nutrition (0-3) +_____	Mwod(+1)
Sleep (hrs) +_____	Stretch(+1)
Stress (0-3)	Yoga(+1)
Tired(0-3)	Nap(+1)
Sore (0-3)	Msg(+1)
Sick (0-3)	Rest(+1)
Injured (0-3)	Ice(+1)
Recovery Factor	Bwork(+1)

THURSDAY   DATE

Hydration (0-3) +_____	Roll(+1)
Nutrition (0-3) +_____	Mwod(+1)
Sleep (hrs) +_____	Stretch(+1)
Stress (0-3)	Yoga(+1)
Tired(0-3)	Nap(+1)
Sore (0-3)	Msg(+1)
Sick (0-3)	Rest(+1)
Injured (0-3)	Ice(+1)
Recovery Factor	Bwork(+1)

WEEKLY LOG

FRIDAY   DATE

Hydration (0-3) +_____	Roll(+1)
Nutrition (0-3) +_____	Mwod(+1)
Sleep (hrs) +_____	Stretch(+1)
Stress (0-3)	Yoga(+1)
Tired(0-3)	Nap(+1)
Sore (0-3)	Msg(+1)
Sick (0-3)	Rest(+1)
Injured (0-3)	Ice(+1)
Recovery Factor	Bwork(+1)

SATURDAY   DATE

Hydration (0-3) +_____	Roll(+1)
Nutrition (0-3) +_____	Mwod(+1)
Sleep (hrs) +_____	Stretch(+1)
Stress (0-3)	Yoga(+1)
Tired(0-3)	Nap(+1)
Sore (0-3)	Msg(+1)
Sick (0-3)	Rest(+1)
Injured (0-3)	Ice(+1)
Recovery Factor	Bwork(+1)

SUNDAY   DATE

Hydration (0-3) +_____	Roll(+1)
Nutrition (0-3) +_____	Mwod(+1)
Sleep (hrs) +_____	Stretch(+1)
Stress (0-3)	Yoga(+1)
Tired(0-3)	Nap(+1)
Sore (0-3)	Msg(+1)
Sick (0-3)	Rest(+1)
Injured (0-3)	Ice(+1)
Recovery Factor	Bwork(+1)

NOTES

Weekly RF Tracking

M _____
T _____
W _____
T _____
F _____
S _____
S _____

Average
Recovery Factor _____

BLOCK _____ CYCLE _____ WEEK _____

MONDAY   DATE

_____

Hydration (0-3) + _____	Roll(+1)
Nutrition (0-3) + _____	Mwod(+1)
Sleep (hrs) + _____	Stretch(+1)
Stress (0-3)	Yoga(+1)
Tired(0-3)	Nap(+1)
Sore (0-3)	Msg(+1)
Sick (0-3)	Rest(+1)
Injured (0-3)	Ice(+1)
Recovery Factor	Bwork(+1)

TUESDAY   DATE

_____

Hydration (0-3) + _____	Roll(+1)
Nutrition (0-3) + _____	Mwod(+1)
Sleep (hrs) + _____	Stretch(+1)
Stress (0-3)	Yoga(+1)
Tired(0-3)	Nap(+1)
Sore (0-3)	Msg(+1)
Sick (0-3)	Rest(+1)
Injured (0-3)	Ice(+1)
Recovery Factor	Bwork(+1)

WEDNESDAY   DATE

_____

Hydration (0-3) + _____	Roll(+1)
Nutrition (0-3) + _____	Mwod(+1)
Sleep (hrs) + _____	Stretch(+1)
Stress (0-3)	Yoga(+1)
Tired(0-3)	Nap(+1)
Sore (0-3)	Msg(+1)
Sick (0-3)	Rest(+1)
Injured (0-3)	Ice(+1)
Recovery Factor	Bwork(+1)

THURSDAY   DATE

_____

Hydration (0-3) + _____	Roll(+1)
Nutrition (0-3) + _____	Mwod(+1)
Sleep (hrs) + _____	Stretch(+1)
Stress (0-3)	Yoga(+1)
Tired(0-3)	Nap(+1)
Sore (0-3)	Msg(+1)
Sick (0-3)	Rest(+1)
Injured (0-3)	Ice(+1)
Recovery Factor	Bwork(+1)

WEEKLY LOG

FRIDAY   DATE

_____

Hydration (0-3) + _____	Roll(+1)
Nutrition (0-3) + _____	Mwod(+1)
Sleep (hrs) + _____	Stretch(+1)
Stress (0-3)	Yoga(+1)
Tired(0-3)	Nap(+1)
Sore (0-3)	Msg(+1)
Sick (0-3)	Rest(+1)
Injured (0-3)	Ice(+1)
Recovery Factor	Bwork(+1)

SATURDAY   DATE

_____

Hydration (0-3) + _____	Roll(+1)
Nutrition (0-3) + _____	Mwod(+1)
Sleep (hrs) + _____	Stretch(+1)
Stress (0-3)	Yoga(+1)
Tired(0-3)	Nap(+1)
Sore (0-3)	Msg(+1)
Sick (0-3)	Rest(+1)
Injured (0-3)	Ice(+1)
Recovery Factor	Bwork(+1)

SUNDAY   DATE

_____

Hydration (0-3) + _____	Roll(+1)
Nutrition (0-3) + _____	Mwod(+1)
Sleep (hrs) + _____	Stretch(+1)
Stress (0-3)	Yoga(+1)
Tired(0-3)	Nap(+1)
Sore (0-3)	Msg(+1)
Sick (0-3)	Rest(+1)
Injured (0-3)	Ice(+1)
Recovery Factor	Bwork(+1)

NOTES

Weekly RF Tracking

M _____
T _____
W _____
T _____
F _____
S _____
S _____
Average
Recovery Factor _____

BLOCK _____ CYCLE _____ WEEK _____

MONDAY   DATE _____

Hydration (0-3) + _____	Roll(+1)
Nutrition (0-3) + _____	Mwod(+1)
Sleep (hrs) + _____	Stretch(+1)
Stress (0-3)	Yoga(+1)
Tired(0-3)	Nap(+1)
Sore (0-3)	Msg(+1)
Sick (0-3)	Rest(+1)
Injured (0-3)	Ice(+1)
Recovery Factor	Bwork(+1)

TUESDAY   DATE _____

Hydration (0-3) + _____	Roll(+1)
Nutrition (0-3) + _____	Mwod(+1)
Sleep (hrs) + _____	Stretch(+1)
Stress (0-3)	Yoga(+1)
Tired(0-3)	Nap(+1)
Sore (0-3)	Msg(+1)
Sick (0-3)	Rest(+1)
Injured (0-3)	Ice(+1)
Recovery Factor	Bwork(+1)

WEDNESDAY   DATE _____

Hydration (0-3) + _____	Roll(+1)
Nutrition (0-3) + _____	Mwod(+1)
Sleep (hrs) + _____	Stretch(+1)
Stress (0-3)	Yoga(+1)
Tired(0-3)	Nap(+1)
Sore (0-3)	Msg(+1)
Sick (0-3)	Rest(+1)
Injured (0-3)	Ice(+1)
Recovery Factor	Bwork(+1)

THURSDAY   DATE _____

Hydration (0-3) + _____	Roll(+1)
Nutrition (0-3) + _____	Mwod(+1)
Sleep (hrs) + _____	Stretch(+1)
Stress (0-3)	Yoga(+1)
Tired(0-3)	Nap(+1)
Sore (0-3)	Msg(+1)
Sick (0-3)	Rest(+1)
Injured (0-3)	Ice(+1)
Recovery Factor	Bwork(+1)

WEEKLY LOG

FRIDAY   DATE

_____

_____

_____

_____

_____

_____

_____

_____

Hydration (0-3)	+_____	Roll(+1)
Nutrition (0-3)	+_____	Mwod(+1)
Sleep (hrs)	+_____	Stretch(+1)
Stress (0-3)		Yoga(+1)
Tired(0-3)		Nap(+1)
Sore (0-3)		Msg(+1)
Sick (0-3)		Rest(+1)
Injured (0-3)		Ice(+1)
Recovery Factor		Bwork(+1)

SATURDAY   DATE

_____

_____

_____

_____

_____

_____

_____

_____

Hydration (0-3)	+_____	Roll(+1)
Nutrition (0-3)	+_____	Mwod(+1)
Sleep (hrs)	+_____	Stretch(+1)
Stress (0-3)		Yoga(+1)
Tired(0-3)		Nap(+1)
Sore (0-3)		Msg(+1)
Sick (0-3)		Rest(+1)
Injured (0-3)		Ice(+1)
Recovery Factor		Bwork(+1)

SUNDAY   DATE

_____

_____

_____

_____

_____

_____

_____

_____

Hydration (0-3)	+_____	Roll(+1)
Nutrition (0-3)	+_____	Mwod(+1)
Sleep (hrs)	+_____	Stretch(+1)
Stress (0-3)		Yoga(+1)
Tired(0-3)		Nap(+1)
Sore (0-3)		Msg(+1)
Sick (0-3)		Rest(+1)
Injured (0-3)		Ice(+1)
Recovery Factor		Bwork(+1)

NOTES

Weekly RF Tracking

M _____

T _____

W _____

T _____

F _____

S _____

S _____

Average
Recovery Factor _____

BLOCK _____ CYCLE _____ WEEK _____

MONDAY   DATE _____

_____

Hydration (0-3) +_____	Roll(+1)
Nutrition (0-3) +_____	Mwod(+1)
Sleep (hrs) +_____	Stretch(+1)
Stress (0-3)	Yoga(+1)
Tired(0-3)	Nap(+1)
Sore (0-3)	Msg(+1)
Sick (0-3)	Rest(+1)
Injured (0-3)	Ice(+1)
Recovery Factor	Bwork(+1)

TUESDAY   DATE _____

_____

Hydration (0-3) +_____	Roll(+1)
Nutrition (0-3) +_____	Mwod(+1)
Sleep (hrs) +_____	Stretch(+1)
Stress (0-3)	Yoga(+1)
Tired(0-3)	Nap(+1)
Sore (0-3)	Msg(+1)
Sick (0-3)	Rest(+1)
Injured (0-3)	Ice(+1)
Recovery Factor	Bwork(+1)

WEDNESDAY   DATE _____

_____

Hydration (0-3) +_____	Roll(+1)
Nutrition (0-3) +_____	Mwod(+1)
Sleep (hrs) +_____	Stretch(+1)
Stress (0-3)	Yoga(+1)
Tired(0-3)	Nap(+1)
Sore (0-3)	Msg(+1)
Sick (0-3)	Rest(+1)
Injured (0-3)	Ice(+1)
Recovery Factor	Bwork(+1)

THURSDAY   DATE _____

_____

Hydration (0-3) +_____	Roll(+1)
Nutrition (0-3) +_____	Mwod(+1)
Sleep (hrs) +_____	Stretch(+1)
Stress (0-3)	Yoga(+1)
Tired(0-3)	Nap(+1)
Sore (0-3)	Msg(+1)
Sick (0-3)	Rest(+1)
Injured (0-3)	Ice(+1)
Recovery Factor	Bwork(+1)

WEEKLY LOG

FRIDAY   DATE

_____

Hydration (0-3) +_____	Roll(+1)
Nutrition (0-3) +_____	Mwod(+1)
Sleep (hrs) +_____	Stretch(+1)
Stress (0-3)	Yoga(+1)
Tired(0-3)	Nap(+1)
Sore (0-3)	Msg(+1)
Sick (0-3)	Rest(+1)
Injured (0-3)	Ice(+1)
Recovery Factor	Bwork(+1)

SATURDAY   DATE

_____

Hydration (0-3) +_____	Roll(+1)
Nutrition (0-3) +_____	Mwod(+1)
Sleep (hrs) +_____	Stretch(+1)
Stress (0-3)	Yoga(+1)
Tired(0-3)	Nap(+1)
Sore (0-3)	Msg(+1)
Sick (0-3)	Rest(+1)
Injured (0-3)	Ice(+1)
Recovery Factor	Bwork(+1)

SUNDAY   DATE

_____

Hydration (0-3) +_____	Roll(+1)
Nutrition (0-3) +_____	Mwod(+1)
Sleep (hrs) +_____	Stretch(+1)
Stress (0-3)	Yoga(+1)
Tired(0-3)	Nap(+1)
Sore (0-3)	Msg(+1)
Sick (0-3)	Rest(+1)
Injured (0-3)	Ice(+1)
Recovery Factor	Bwork(+1)

NOTES

Weekly RF Tracking

M _____
T _____
W _____
T _____
F _____
S _____
S _____
Average
Recovery Factor _____

BLOCK _____ CYCLE _____ WEEK _____

MONDAY   DATE

Hydration (0-3) +_____	Roll(+1)
Nutrition (0-3) +_____	Mwod(+1)
Sleep (hrs) +_____	Stretch(+1)
Stress (0-3)	Yoga(+1)
Tired(0-3)	Nap(+1)
Sore (0-3)	Msg(+1)
Sick (0-3)	Rest(+1)
Injured (0-3)	Ice(+1)
Recovery Factor	Bwork(+1)

TUESDAY   DATE

Hydration (0-3) +_____	Roll(+1)
Nutrition (0-3) +_____	Mwod(+1)
Sleep (hrs) +_____	Stretch(+1)
Stress (0-3)	Yoga(+1)
Tired(0-3)	Nap(+1)
Sore (0-3)	Msg(+1)
Sick (0-3)	Rest(+1)
Injured (0-3)	Ice(+1)
Recovery Factor	Bwork(+1)

WEDNESDAY   DATE

Hydration (0-3) +_____	Roll(+1)
Nutrition (0-3) +_____	Mwod(+1)
Sleep (hrs) +_____	Stretch(+1)
Stress (0-3)	Yoga(+1)
Tired(0-3)	Nap(+1)
Sore (0-3)	Msg(+1)
Sick (0-3)	Rest(+1)
Injured (0-3)	Ice(+1)
Recovery Factor	Bwork(+1)

THURSDAY   DATE

Hydration (0-3) +_____	Roll(+1)
Nutrition (0-3) +_____	Mwod(+1)
Sleep (hrs) +_____	Stretch(+1)
Stress (0-3)	Yoga(+1)
Tired(0-3)	Nap(+1)
Sore (0-3)	Msg(+1)
Sick (0-3)	Rest(+1)
Injured (0-3)	Ice(+1)
Recovery Factor	Bwork(+1)

WEEKLY LOG

FRIDAY   **DATE** _____

_____

_____

_____

_____

_____

_____

_____

_____

_____

Hydration (0-3) + _____	Roll(+1)
Nutrition (0-3) + _____	Mwod(+1)
Sleep (hrs) + _____	Stretch(+1)
Stress (0-3)	Yoga(+1)
Tired(0-3)	Nap(+1)
Sore (0-3)	Msg(+1)
Sick (0-3)	Rest(+1)
Injured (0-3)	Ice(+1)
Recovery Factor	Bwork(+1)

SATURDAY   **DATE** _____

_____

_____

_____

_____

_____

_____

_____

_____

Hydration (0-3) + _____	Roll(+1)
Nutrition (0-3) + _____	Mwod(+1)
Sleep (hrs) + _____	Stretch(+1)
Stress (0-3)	Yoga(+1)
Tired(0-3)	Nap(+1)
Sore (0-3)	Msg(+1)
Sick (0-3)	Rest(+1)
Injured (0-3)	Ice(+1)
Recovery Factor	Bwork(+1)

SUNDAY   **DATE** _____

_____

_____

_____

_____

_____

_____

_____

_____

Hydration (0-3) + _____	Roll(+1)
Nutrition (0-3) + _____	Mwod(+1)
Sleep (hrs) + _____	Stretch(+1)
Stress (0-3)	Yoga(+1)
Tired(0-3)	Nap(+1)
Sore (0-3)	Msg(+1)
Sick (0-3)	Rest(+1)
Injured (0-3)	Ice(+1)
Recovery Factor	Bwork(+1)

NOTES

Weekly RF Tracking

M _____

T _____

W _____

T _____

F _____

S _____

S _____

Average
Recovery Factor _____

BLOCK _____ CYCLE _____ WEEK _____

MONDAY   DATE _____

_____
_____
_____
_____
_____
_____
_____
_____

Hydration (0-3) +_____ Roll(+1)
Nutrition (0-3) +_____ Mwod(+1)
Sleep (hrs)   +_____ Stretch(+1)
Stress (0-3)   Yoga(+1)
Tired(0-3)   Nap(+1)
Sore (0-3)   Msg(+1)
Sick (0-3)   Rest(+1)
Injured (0-3)   Ice(+1)
Recovery Factor   Bwork(+1)

TUESDAY   DATE _____

_____
_____
_____
_____
_____
_____
_____
_____

Hydration (0-3) +_____ Roll(+1)
Nutrition (0-3) +_____ Mwod(+1)
Sleep (hrs)   +_____ Stretch(+1)
Stress (0-3)   Yoga(+1)
Tired(0-3)   Nap(+1)
Sore (0-3)   Msg(+1)
Sick (0-3)   Rest(+1)
Injured (0-3)   Ice(+1)
Recovery Factor   Bwork(+1)

WEDNESDAY   DATE _____

_____
_____
_____
_____
_____
_____
_____
_____

Hydration (0-3) +_____ Roll(+1)
Nutrition (0-3) +_____ Mwod(+1)
Sleep (hrs)   +_____ Stretch(+1)
Stress (0-3)   Yoga(+1)
Tired(0-3)   Nap(+1)
Sore (0-3)   Msg(+1)
Sick (0-3)   Rest(+1)
Injured (0-3)   Ice(+1)
Recovery Factor   Bwork(+1)

THURSDAY   DATE _____

_____
_____
_____
_____
_____
_____
_____
_____

Hydration (0-3) +_____ Roll(+1)
Nutrition (0-3) +_____ Mwod(+1)
Sleep (hrs)   +_____ Stretch(+1)
Stress (0-3)   Yoga(+1)
Tired(0-3)   Nap(+1)
Sore (0-3)   Msg(+1)
Sick (0-3)   Rest(+1)
Injured (0-3)   Ice(+1)
Recovery Factor   Bwork(+1)

WEEKLY LOG

FRIDAY   **DATE**

_____

_____

_____

_____

_____

_____

_____

_____

Hydration (0-3) +_____	Roll(+1)
Nutrition (0-3) +_____	Mwod(+1)
Sleep (hrs) +_____	Stretch(+1)
Stress (0-3)	Yoga(+1)
Tired(0-3)	Nap(+1)
Sore (0-3)	Msg(+1)
Sick (0-3)	Rest(+1)
Injured (0-3)	Ice(+1)
Recovery Factor	Bwork(+1)

SATURDAY   **DATE**

_____

_____

_____

_____

_____

_____

_____

_____

Hydration (0-3) +_____	Roll(+1)
Nutrition (0-3) +_____	Mwod(+1)
Sleep (hrs) +_____	Stretch(+1)
Stress (0-3)	Yoga(+1)
Tired(0-3)	Nap(+1)
Sore (0-3)	Msg(+1)
Sick (0-3)	Rest(+1)
Injured (0-3)	Ice(+1)
Recovery Factor	Bwork(+1)

SUNDAY   **DATE**

_____

_____

_____

_____

_____

_____

_____

_____

Hydration (0-3) +_____	Roll(+1)
Nutrition (0-3) +_____	Mwod(+1)
Sleep (hrs) +_____	Stretch(+1)
Stress (0-3)	Yoga(+1)
Tired(0-3)	Nap(+1)
Sore (0-3)	Msg(+1)
Sick (0-3)	Rest(+1)
Injured (0-3)	Ice(+1)
Recovery Factor	Bwork(+1)

NOTES

Weekly RF Tracking

M _____

T _____

W _____

T _____

F _____

S _____

S _____

Average
Recovery Factor _____

BLOCK _____ CYCLE _____ WEEK _____

MONDAY   DATE

Hydration (0-3) + _____		Roll(+1)
Nutrition (0-3) + _____		Mwod(+1)
Sleep (hrs)	+ _____	Stretch(+1)
Stress (0-3)		Yoga(+1)
Tired(0-3)		Nap(+1)
Sore (0-3)		Msg(+1)
Sick (0-3)		Rest(+1)
Injured (0-3)		Ice(+1)
Recovery Factor		Bwork(+1)

TUESDAY   DATE

Hydration (0-3) + _____		Roll(+1)
Nutrition (0-3) + _____		Mwod(+1)
Sleep (hrs)	+ _____	Stretch(+1)
Stress (0-3)		Yoga(+1)
Tired(0-3)		Nap(+1)
Sore (0-3)		Msg(+1)
Sick (0-3)		Rest(+1)
Injured (0-3)		Ice(+1)
Recovery Factor		Bwork(+1)

WEDNESDAY   DATE

Hydration (0-3) + _____		Roll(+1)
Nutrition (0-3) + _____		Mwod(+1)
Sleep (hrs)	+ _____	Stretch(+1)
Stress (0-3)		Yoga(+1)
Tired(0-3)		Nap(+1)
Sore (0-3)		Msg(+1)
Sick (0-3)		Rest(+1)
Injured (0-3)		Ice(+1)
Recovery Factor		Bwork(+1)

THURSDAY   DATE

Hydration (0-3) + _____		Roll(+1)
Nutrition (0-3) + _____		Mwod(+1)
Sleep (hrs)	+ _____	Stretch(+1)
Stress (0-3)		Yoga(+1)
Tired(0-3)		Nap(+1)
Sore (0-3)		Msg(+1)
Sick (0-3)		Rest(+1)
Injured (0-3)		Ice(+1)
Recovery Factor		Bwork(+1)

WEEKLY LOG

FRIDAY   **DATE**

_____

Hydration (0-3) +_____ Roll(+1)
Nutrition (0-3) +_____ Mwod(+1)
Sleep (hrs)   +_____ Stretch(+1)
Stress (0-3)   -   Yoga(+1)
Tired(0-3)   -   Nap(+1)
Sore (0-3)   -   Msg(+1)
Sick (0-3)   -   Rest(+1)
Injured (0-3)   -   Ice(+1)
Recovery Factor   Bwork(+1)

SATURDAY   **DATE**

_____

Hydration (0-3) +_____ Roll(+1)
Nutrition (0-3) +_____ Mwod(+1)
Sleep (hrs)   +_____ Stretch(+1)
Stress (0-3)   -   Yoga(+1)
Tired(0-3)   -   Nap(+1)
Sore (0-3)   -   Msg(+1)
Sick (0-3)   -   Rest(+1)
Injured (0-3)   -   Ice(+1)
Recovery Factor   Bwork(+1)

SUNDAY   **DATE**

_____

Hydration (0-3) +_____ Roll(+1)
Nutrition (0-3) +_____ Mwod(+1)
Sleep (hrs)   +_____ Stretch(+1)
Stress (0-3)   -   Yoga(+1)
Tired(0-3)   -   Nap(+1)
Sore (0-3)   -   Msg(+1)
Sick (0-3)   -   Rest(+1)
Injured (0-3)   -   Ice(+1)
Recovery Factor   Bwork(+1)

NOTES

Weekly RF Tracking
M _____
T _____
W _____
T _____
F _____
S _____
S _____
Average
Recovery Factor _____

BLOCK _____ CYCLE _____ WEEK _____

MONDAY   DATE _____

_____
_____
_____
_____
_____
_____
_____
_____
_____

Hydration (0-3) +_____		Roll(+1)
Nutrition (0-3) +_____		Mwod(+1)
Sleep (hrs) +_____		Stretch(+1)
Stress (0-3)		Yoga(+1)
Tired(0-3)		Nap(+1)
Sore (0-3)		Msg(+1)
Sick (0-3)		Rest(+1)
Injured (0-3)		Ice(+1)
Recovery Factor		Bwork(+1)

TUESDAY   DATE _____

_____
_____
_____
_____
_____
_____
_____
_____
_____

Hydration (0-3) +_____		Roll(+1)
Nutrition (0-3) +_____		Mwod(+1)
Sleep (hrs) +_____		Stretch(+1)
Stress (0-3)		Yoga(+1)
Tired(0-3)		Nap(+1)
Sore (0-3)		Msg(+1)
Sick (0-3)		Rest(+1)
Injured (0-3)		Ice(+1)
Recovery Factor		Bwork(+1)

WEDNESDAY   DATE _____

_____
_____
_____
_____
_____
_____
_____
_____
_____

Hydration (0-3) +_____		Roll(+1)
Nutrition (0-3) +_____		Mwod(+1)
Sleep (hrs) +_____		Stretch(+1)
Stress (0-3)		Yoga(+1)
Tired(0-3)		Nap(+1)
Sore (0-3)		Msg(+1)
Sick (0-3)		Rest(+1)
Injured (0-3)		Ice(+1)
Recovery Factor		Bwork(+1)

THURSDAY   DATE _____

_____
_____
_____
_____
_____
_____
_____
_____
_____

Hydration (0-3) +_____		Roll(+1)
Nutrition (0-3) +_____		Mwod(+1)
Sleep (hrs) +_____		Stretch(+1)
Stress (0-3)		Yoga(+1)
Tired(0-3)		Nap(+1)
Sore (0-3)		Msg(+1)
Sick (0-3)		Rest(+1)
Injured (0-3)		Ice(+1)
Recovery Factor		Bwork(+1)

WEEKLY LOG

FRIDAY   DATE

_____

Hydration (0-3) +_____ Roll(+1)
Nutrition (0-3) +_____ Mwod(+1)
Sleep (hrs) +_____ Stretch(+1)
Stress (0-3) Yoga(+1)
Tired(0-3) Nap(+1)
Sore (0-3) Msg(+1)
Sick (0-3) Rest(+1)
Injured (0-3) Ice(+1)
Recovery Factor Bwork(+1)

SATURDAY   DATE

_____

Hydration (0-3) +_____ Roll(+1)
Nutrition (0-3) +_____ Mwod(+1)
Sleep (hrs) +_____ Stretch(+1)
Stress (0-3) Yoga(+1)
Tired(0-3) Nap(+1)
Sore (0-3) Msg(+1)
Sick (0-3) Rest(+1)
Injured (0-3) Ice(+1)
Recovery Factor Bwork(+1)

SUNDAY   DATE

_____

Hydration (0-3) +_____ Roll(+1)
Nutrition (0-3) +_____ Mwod(+1)
Sleep (hrs) +_____ Stretch(+1)
Stress (0-3) Yoga(+1)
Tired(0-3) Nap(+1)
Sore (0-3) Msg(+1)
Sick (0-3) Rest(+1)
Injured (0-3) Ice(+1)
Recovery Factor Bwork(+1)

NOTES

Weekly RF Tracking
M _____
T _____
W _____
T _____
F _____
S _____
S _____
Average
Recovery Factor _____

BLOCK _____ CYCLE _____ WEEK _____

MONDAY   DATE _____

_____	Hydration (0-3) + _____	Roll(+1)
_____	Nutrition (0-3) + _____	Mwod(+1)
_____	Sleep (hrs) + _____	Stretch(+1)
_____	Stress (0-3)	Yoga(+1)
_____	Tired(0-3)	Nap(+1)
_____	Sore (0-3)	Msg(+1)
_____	Sick (0-3)	Rest(+1)
_____	Injured (0-3)	Ice(+1)
_____	Recovery Factor	Bwork(+1)

TUESDAY   DATE _____

_____	Hydration (0-3) + _____	Roll(+1)
_____	Nutrition (0-3) + _____	Mwod(+1)
_____	Sleep (hrs) + _____	Stretch(+1)
_____	Stress (0-3)	Yoga(+1)
_____	Tired(0-3)	Nap(+1)
_____	Sore (0-3)	Msg(+1)
_____	Sick (0-3)	Rest(+1)
_____	Injured (0-3)	Ice(+1)
_____	Recovery Factor	Bwork(+1)

WEDNESDAY   DATE _____

_____	Hydration (0-3) + _____	Roll(+1)
_____	Nutrition (0-3) + _____	Mwod(+1)
_____	Sleep (hrs) + _____	Stretch(+1)
_____	Stress (0-3)	Yoga(+1)
_____	Tired(0-3)	Nap(+1)
_____	Sore (0-3)	Msg(+1)
_____	Sick (0-3)	Rest(+1)
_____	Injured (0-3)	Ice(+1)
_____	Recovery Factor	Bwork(+1)

THURSDAY   DATE _____

_____	Hydration (0-3) + _____	Roll(+1)
_____	Nutrition (0-3) + _____	Mwod(+1)
_____	Sleep (hrs) + _____	Stretch(+1)
_____	Stress (0-3)	Yoga(+1)
_____	Tired(0-3)	Nap(+1)
_____	Sore (0-3)	Msg(+1)
_____	Sick (0-3)	Rest(+1)
_____	Injured (0-3)	Ice(+1)
_____	Recovery Factor	Bwork(+1)

WEEKLY LOG

FRIDAY   DATE

_____

Hydration (0-3) +_____ Roll(+1)
Nutrition (0-3) +_____ Mwod(+1)
Sleep (hrs)   +_____ Stretch(+1)
Stress (0-3)   Yoga(+1)
Tired(0-3)   Nap(+1)
Sore (0-3)   Msg(+1)
Sick (0-3)   Rest(+1)
Injured (0-3)   Ice(+1)
Recovery Factor   Bwork(+1)

SATURDAY   DATE

_____

Hydration (0-3) +_____ Roll(+1)
Nutrition (0-3) +_____ Mwod(+1)
Sleep (hrs)   +_____ Stretch(+1)
Stress (0-3)   Yoga(+1)
Tired(0-3)   Nap(+1)
Sore (0-3)   Msg(+1)
Sick (0-3)   Rest(+1)
Injured (0-3)   Ice(+1)
Recovery Factor   Bwork(+1)

SUNDAY   DATE

_____

Hydration (0-3) +_____ Roll(+1)
Nutrition (0-3) +_____ Mwod(+1)
Sleep (hrs)   +_____ Stretch(+1)
Stress (0-3)   Yoga(+1)
Tired(0-3)   Nap(+1)
Sore (0-3)   Msg(+1)
Sick (0-3)   Rest(+1)
Injured (0-3)   Ice(+1)
Recovery Factor   Bwork(+1)

NOTES

Weekly RF Tracking
M _____
T _____
W _____
T _____
F _____
S _____
S _____
Average
Recovery Factor _____

BLOCK _____ CYCLE _____ WEEK _____

MONDAY   DATE

_____

Hydration (0-3) +_____	Roll(+1)
Nutrition (0-3) +_____	Mwod(+1)
Sleep (hrs) +_____	Stretch(+1)
Stress (0-3)	Yoga(+1)
Tired(0-3)	Nap(+1)
Sore (0-3)	Msg(+1)
Sick (0-3)	Rest(+1)
Injured (0-3)	Ice(+1)
Recovery Factor	Bwork(+1)

TUESDAY   DATE

_____

Hydration (0-3) +_____	Roll(+1)
Nutrition (0-3) +_____	Mwod(+1)
Sleep (hrs) +_____	Stretch(+1)
Stress (0-3)	Yoga(+1)
Tired(0-3)	Nap(+1)
Sore (0-3)	Msg(+1)
Sick (0-3)	Rest(+1)
Injured (0-3)	Ice(+1)
Recovery Factor	Bwork(+1)

WEDNESDAY   DATE

_____

Hydration (0-3) +_____	Roll(+1)
Nutrition (0-3) +_____	Mwod(+1)
Sleep (hrs) +_____	Stretch(+1)
Stress (0-3)	Yoga(+1)
Tired(0-3)	Nap(+1)
Sore (0-3)	Msg(+1)
Sick (0-3)	Rest(+1)
Injured (0-3)	Ice(+1)
Recovery Factor	Bwork(+1)

THURSDAY   DATE

_____

Hydration (0-3) +_____	Roll(+1)
Nutrition (0-3) +_____	Mwod(+1)
Sleep (hrs) +_____	Stretch(+1)
Stress (0-3)	Yoga(+1)
Tired(0-3)	Nap(+1)
Sore (0-3)	Msg(+1)
Sick (0-3)	Rest(+1)
Injured (0-3)	Ice(+1)
Recovery Factor	Bwork(+1)

WEEKLY LOG

FRIDAY   DATE

_____

_____

_____

_____

_____

_____

_____

_____

_____

Hydration (0-3) +_____	Roll(+1)
Nutrition (0-3) +_____	Mwod(+1)
Sleep (hrs) +_____	Stretch(+1)
Stress (0-3)	Yoga(+1)
Tired(0-3)	Nap(+1)
Sore (0-3)	Msg(+1)
Sick (0-3)	Rest(+1)
Injured (0-3)	Ice(+1)
Recovery Factor	Bwork(+1)

SATURDAY   DATE

_____

_____

_____

_____

_____

_____

_____

_____

_____

Hydration (0-3) +_____	Roll(+1)
Nutrition (0-3) +_____	Mwod(+1)
Sleep (hrs) +_____	Stretch(+1)
Stress (0-3)	Yoga(+1)
Tired(0-3)	Nap(+1)
Sore (0-3)	Msg(+1)
Sick (0-3)	Rest(+1)
Injured (0-3)	Ice(+1)
Recovery Factor	Bwork(+1)

SUNDAY   DATE

_____

_____

_____

_____

_____

_____

_____

_____

_____

Hydration (0-3) +_____	Roll(+1)
Nutrition (0-3) +_____	Mwod(+1)
Sleep (hrs) +_____	Stretch(+1)
Stress (0-3)	Yoga(+1)
Tired(0-3)	Nap(+1)
Sore (0-3)	Msg(+1)
Sick (0-3)	Rest(+1)
Injured (0-3)	Ice(+1)
Recovery Factor	Bwork(+1)

NOTES

Weekly RF Tracking

M _____

T _____

W _____

T _____

F _____

S _____

S _____

Average
Recovery Factor _____

BLOCK _____ CYCLE _____ WEEK _____

MONDAY   DATE _____

_____ Hydration (0-3) +_____ Roll(+1)
_____ Nutrition (0-3) +_____ Mwod(+1)
_____ Sleep (hrs)   +_____ Stretch(+1)
_____ Stress (0-3) ____ Yoga(+1)
_____ Tired(0-3)   ____ Nap(+1)
_____ Sore (0-3)   ____ Msg(+1)
_____ Sick (0-3)   ____ Rest(+1)
_____ Injured (0-3) ____ Ice(+1)
_____ Recovery Factor   Bwork(+1)

TUESDAY   DATE _____

_____ Hydration (0-3) +_____ Roll(+1)
_____ Nutrition (0-3) +_____ Mwod(+1)
_____ Sleep (hrs)   +_____ Stretch(+1)
_____ Stress (0-3) ____ Yoga(+1)
_____ Tired(0-3)   ____ Nap(+1)
_____ Sore (0-3)   ____ Msg(+1)
_____ Sick (0-3)   ____ Rest(+1)
_____ Injured (0-3) ____ Ice(+1)
_____ Recovery Factor   Bwork(+1)

WEDNESDAY   DATE _____

_____ Hydration (0-3) +_____ Roll(+1)
_____ Nutrition (0-3) +_____ Mwod(+1)
_____ Sleep (hrs)   +_____ Stretch(+1)
_____ Stress (0-3) ____ Yoga(+1)
_____ Tired(0-3)   ____ Nap(+1)
_____ Sore (0-3)   ____ Msg(+1)
_____ Sick (0-3)   ____ Rest(+1)
_____ Injured (0-3) ____ Ice(+1)
_____ Recovery Factor   Bwork(+1)

THURSDAY   DATE _____

_____ Hydration (0-3) +_____ Roll(+1)
_____ Nutrition (0-3) +_____ Mwod(+1)
_____ Sleep (hrs)   +_____ Stretch(+1)
_____ Stress (0-3) ____ Yoga(+1)
_____ Tired(0-3)   ____ Nap(+1)
_____ Sore (0-3)   ____ Msg(+1)
_____ Sick (0-3)   ____ Rest(+1)
_____ Injured (0-3) ____ Ice(+1)
_____ Recovery Factor   Bwork(+1)

WEEKLY LOG

FRIDAY   DATE

_____

_____

_____

_____

_____

_____

_____

_____

_____

Hydration (0-3) + _____		Roll(+1)
Nutrition (0-3) + _____		Mwod(+1)
Sleep (hrs) + _____		Stretch(+1)
Stress (0-3)		Yoga(+1)
Tired(0-3)		Nap(+1)
Sore (0-3)		Msg(+1)
Sick (0-3)		Rest(+1)
Injured (0-3)		Ice(+1)
Recovery Factor		Bwork(+1)

SATURDAY   DATE

_____

_____

_____

_____

_____

_____

_____

_____

_____

Hydration (0-3) + _____		Roll(+1)
Nutrition (0-3) + _____		Mwod(+1)
Sleep (hrs) + _____		Stretch(+1)
Stress (0-3)		Yoga(+1)
Tired(0-3)		Nap(+1)
Sore (0-3)		Msg(+1)
Sick (0-3)		Rest(+1)
Injured (0-3)		Ice(+1)
Recovery Factor		Bwork(+1)

SUNDAY   DATE

_____

_____

_____

_____

_____

_____

_____

_____

_____

Hydration (0-3) + _____		Roll(+1)
Nutrition (0-3) + _____		Mwod(+1)
Sleep (hrs) + _____		Stretch(+1)
Stress (0-3)		Yoga(+1)
Tired(0-3)		Nap(+1)
Sore (0-3)		Msg(+1)
Sick (0-3)		Rest(+1)
Injured (0-3)		Ice(+1)
Recovery Factor		Bwork(+1)

NOTES

Weekly RF Tracking

M _____

T _____

W _____

T _____

F _____

S _____

S _____

Average
Recovery Factor _____

BLOCK _____ CYCLE _____ WEEK _____

MONDAY   DATE

Hydration (0-3) +_____	Roll(+1)
Nutrition (0-3) +_____	Mwod(+1)
Sleep (hrs) +_____	Stretch(+1)
Stress (0-3)	Yoga(+1)
Tired(0-3)	Nap(+1)
Sore (0-3)	Msg(+1)
Sick (0-3)	Rest(+1)
Injured (0-3)	Ice(+1)
Recovery Factor	Bwork(+1)

TUESDAY   DATE

Hydration (0-3) +_____	Roll(+1)
Nutrition (0-3) +_____	Mwod(+1)
Sleep (hrs) +_____	Stretch(+1)
Stress (0-3)	Yoga(+1)
Tired(0-3)	Nap(+1)
Sore (0-3)	Msg(+1)
Sick (0-3)	Rest(+1)
Injured (0-3)	Ice(+1)
Recovery Factor	Bwork(+1)

WEDNESDAY   DATE

Hydration (0-3) +_____	Roll(+1)
Nutrition (0-3) +_____	Mwod(+1)
Sleep (hrs) +_____	Stretch(+1)
Stress (0-3)	Yoga(+1)
Tired(0-3)	Nap(+1)
Sore (0-3)	Msg(+1)
Sick (0-3)	Rest(+1)
Injured (0-3)	Ice(+1)
Recovery Factor	Bwork(+1)

THURSDAY   DATE

Hydration (0-3) +_____	Roll(+1)
Nutrition (0-3) +_____	Mwod(+1)
Sleep (hrs) +_____	Stretch(+1)
Stress (0-3)	Yoga(+1)
Tired(0-3)	Nap(+1)
Sore (0-3)	Msg(+1)
Sick (0-3)	Rest(+1)
Injured (0-3)	Ice(+1)
Recovery Factor	Bwork(+1)

WEEKLY LOG

FRIDAY   **DATE**

_____

Hydration (0-3)	+_____	Roll(+1)
Nutrition (0-3)	+_____	Mwod(+1)
Sleep (hrs)	+_____	Stretch(+1)
Stress (0-3)		Yoga(+1)
Tired(0-3)		Nap(+1)
Sore (0-3)		Msg(+1)
Sick (0-3)		Rest(+1)
Injured (0-3)		Ice(+1)
Recovery Factor		Bwork(+1)

SATURDAY   **DATE**

_____

Hydration (0-3)	+_____	Roll(+1)
Nutrition (0-3)	+_____	Mwod(+1)
Sleep (hrs)	+_____	Stretch(+1)
Stress (0-3)		Yoga(+1)
Tired(0-3)		Nap(+1)
Sore (0-3)		Msg(+1)
Sick (0-3)		Rest(+1)
Injured (0-3)		Ice(+1)
Recovery Factor		Bwork(+1)

SUNDAY   **DATE**

_____

Hydration (0-3)	+_____	Roll(+1)
Nutrition (0-3)	+_____	Mwod(+1)
Sleep (hrs)	+_____	Stretch(+1)
Stress (0-3)		Yoga(+1)
Tired(0-3)		Nap(+1)
Sore (0-3)		Msg(+1)
Sick (0-3)		Rest(+1)
Injured (0-3)		Ice(+1)
Recovery Factor		Bwork(+1)

NOTES

Weekly RF Tracking

M _____
T _____
W _____
T _____
F _____
S _____
S _____
Average
Recovery Factor _____

BLOCK _____ CYCLE _____ WEEK _____

MONDAY   DATE _____

_____	
_____	Hydration (0-3) +_____ Roll(+1)
_____	Nutrition (0-3) +_____ Mwod(+1)
_____	Sleep (hrs) +_____ Stretch(+1)
_____	Stress (0-3) Yoga(+1)
_____	Tired(0-3) Nap(+1)
_____	Sore (0-3) Msg(+1)
_____	Sick (0-3) Rest(+1)
_____	Injured (0-3) Ice(+1)
_____	Recovery Factor Bwork(+1)

TUESDAY   DATE _____

_____	
_____	Hydration (0-3) +_____ Roll(+1)
_____	Nutrition (0-3) +_____ Mwod(+1)
_____	Sleep (hrs) +_____ Stretch(+1)
_____	Stress (0-3) Yoga(+1)
_____	Tired(0-3) Nap(+1)
_____	Sore (0-3) Msg(+1)
_____	Sick (0-3) Rest(+1)
_____	Injured (0-3) Ice(+1)
_____	Recovery Factor Bwork(+1)

WEDNESDAY   DATE _____

_____	
_____	Hydration (0-3) +_____ Roll(+1)
_____	Nutrition (0-3) +_____ Mwod(+1)
_____	Sleep (hrs) +_____ Stretch(+1)
_____	Stress (0-3) Yoga(+1)
_____	Tired(0-3) Nap(+1)
_____	Sore (0-3) Msg(+1)
_____	Sick (0-3) Rest(+1)
_____	Injured (0-3) Ice(+1)
_____	Recovery Factor Bwork(+1)

THURSDAY   DATE _____

_____	
_____	Hydration (0-3) +_____ Roll(+1)
_____	Nutrition (0-3) +_____ Mwod(+1)
_____	Sleep (hrs) +_____ Stretch(+1)
_____	Stress (0-3) Yoga(+1)
_____	Tired(0-3) Nap(+1)
_____	Sore (0-3) Msg(+1)
_____	Sick (0-3) Rest(+1)
_____	Injured (0-3) Ice(+1)
_____	Recovery Factor Bwork(+1)

WEEKLY LOG

FRIDAY   DATE

_____

Hydration (0-3) +_____	Roll(+1)
Nutrition (0-3) +_____	Mwod(+1)
Sleep (hrs) +_____	Stretch(+1)
Stress (0-3)	Yoga(+1)
Tired(0-3)	Nap(+1)
Sore (0-3)	Msg(+1)
Sick (0-3)	Rest(+1)
Injured (0-3)	Ice(+1)
Recovery Factor	Bwork(+1)

SATURDAY   DATE

_____

Hydration (0-3) +_____	Roll(+1)
Nutrition (0-3) +_____	Mwod(+1)
Sleep (hrs) +_____	Stretch(+1)
Stress (0-3)	Yoga(+1)
Tired(0-3)	Nap(+1)
Sore (0-3)	Msg(+1)
Sick (0-3)	Rest(+1)
Injured (0-3)	Ice(+1)
Recovery Factor	Bwork(+1)

SUNDAY   DATE

_____

Hydration (0-3) +_____	Roll(+1)
Nutrition (0-3) +_____	Mwod(+1)
Sleep (hrs) +_____	Stretch(+1)
Stress (0-3)	Yoga(+1)
Tired(0-3)	Nap(+1)
Sore (0-3)	Msg(+1)
Sick (0-3)	Rest(+1)
Injured (0-3)	Ice(+1)
Recovery Factor	Bwork(+1)

NOTES

Weekly RF Tracking

M _____
T _____
W _____
T _____
F _____
S _____
S _____
Average
Recovery Factor _____

MAX EFFORT TEMPLATE

Set/%	DATE	DATE	DATE	DATE	DATE	DATE	DATE	DATE

Back Squat

Set/%	DATE	DATE	DATE	DATE	DATE	DATE	DATE	DATE

MAX EFFORT TEMPLATE

Set/%	DATE	DATE	DATE	DATE	DATE	DATE	DATE	DATE

Front Squat

Set/%	DATE	DATE	DATE	DATE	DATE	DATE	DATE	DATE

MAX EFFORT TEMPLATE

Set/%	DATE	DATE	DATE	DATE	DATE	DATE	DATE	DATE

Overhead Squat

Set/%	DATE	DATE	DATE	DATE	DATE	DATE	DATE	DATE

MAX EFFORT TEMPLATE

Set/%	DATE	DATE	DATE	DATE	DATE	DATE	DATE	DATE

Deadlift

Set/%	DATE	DATE	DATE	DATE	DATE	DATE	DATE	DATE

MAX EFFORT TEMPLATE

Set/%	DATE	DATE	DATE	DATE	DATE	DATE	DATE	DATE

Clean

Set/%	DATE	DATE	DATE	DATE	DATE	DATE	DATE	DATE

MAX EFFORT TEMPLATE

Set/%	DATE	DATE	DATE	DATE	DATE	DATE	DATE	DATE

Power Clean

Set/%	DATE	DATE	DATE	DATE	DATE	DATE	DATE	DATE

MAX EFFORT TEMPLATE

Set/%	DATE	DATE	DATE	DATE	DATE	DATE	DATE	DATE

Snatch

Set/%	DATE	DATE	DATE	DATE	DATE	DATE	DATE	DATE

MAX EFFORT TEMPLATE

Set/%	DATE	DATE	DATE	DATE	DATE	DATE	DATE	DATE

Power Snatch

Set/%	DATE	DATE	DATE	DATE	DATE	DATE	DATE	DATE

MAX EFFORT TEMPLATE

Set/%	DATE	DATE	DATE	DATE	DATE	DATE	DATE	DATE

Overhead Press

Set/%	DATE	DATE	DATE	DATE	DATE	DATE	DATE	DATE

MAX EFFORT TEMPLATE

Set/%	DATE	DATE	DATE	DATE	DATE	DATE	DATE	DATE

Push Press

Set/%	DATE	DATE	DATE	DATE	DATE	DATE	DATE	DATE

MAX EFFORT TEMPLATE

Set/%	DATE	DATE	DATE	DATE	DATE	DATE	DATE	DATE

Push/Split Jerk

Set/%	DATE	DATE	DATE	DATE	DATE	DATE	DATE	DATE

MAX EFFORT TEMPLATE

Set/%	DATE	DATE	DATE	DATE	DATE	DATE	DATE	DATE

Bench Press

Set/%	DATE	DATE	DATE	DATE	DATE	DATE	DATE	DATE

BENCHMARK WORKOUT LOG

NAME	RX	Load/Scale	Time/Round

NAME	RX	Load/Scale	Time/Round

NAME	RX	Load/Scale	Time/Round

NAME	RX	Load/Scale	Time/Round

BENCHMARK WORKOUT LOG

Load/Scale	Time/Round	Load/Scale	Time/Round	Load/Scale	Time/Round

Load/Scale	Time/Round	Load/Scale	Time/Round	Load/Scale	Time/Round

Load/Scale	Time/Round	Load/Scale	Time/Round	Load/Scale	Time/Round

Load/Scale	Time/Round	Load/Scale	Time/Round	Load/Scale	Time/Round

BENCHMARK WORKOUT LOG

NAME		RX	Load/Scale	Time/Round

NAME		RX	Load/Scale	Time/Round

NAME		RX	Load/Scale	Time/Round

NAME		RX	Load/Scale	Time/Round

BENCHMARK WORKOUT LOG

Load/Scale	Time/Round	Load/Scale	Time/Round	Load/Scale	Time/Round

Load/Scale	Time/Round	Load/Scale	Time/Round	Load/Scale	Time/Round

Load/Scale	Time/Round	Load/Scale	Time/Round	Load/Scale	Time/Round

Load/Scale	Time/Round	Load/Scale	Time/Round	Load/Scale	Time/Round

BENCHMARK WORKOUT LOG

NAME		RX	Load/Scale	Time/Round

NAME		RX	Load/Scale	Time/Round

NAME		RX	Load/Scale	Time/Round

NAME		RX	Load/Scale	Time/Round

BENCHMARK WORKOUT LOG

Load/Scale	Time/Round	Load/Scale	Time/Round	Load/Scale	Time/Round

Load/Scale	Time/Round	Load/Scale	Time/Round	Load/Scale	Time/Round

Load/Scale	Time/Round	Load/Scale	Time/Round	Load/Scale	Time/Round

Load/Scale	Time/Round	Load/Scale	Time/Round	Load/Scale	Time/Round

BENCHMARK WORKOUT LOG

NAME	RX	Load/Scale	Time/Round

NAME	RX	Load/Scale	Time/Round

NAME	RX	Load/Scale	Time/Round

NAME	RX	Load/Scale	Time/Round

BENCHMARK WORKOUT LOG

Load/Scale	Time/Round	Load/Scale	Time/Round	Load/Scale	Time/Round

Load/Scale	Time/Round	Load/Scale	Time/Round	Load/Scale	Time/Round

Load/Scale	Time/Round	Load/Scale	Time/Round	Load/Scale	Time/Round

Load/Scale	Time/Round	Load/Scale	Time/Round	Load/Scale	Time/Round

BENCHMARK WORKOUT LOG

NAME	RX	Load/Scale	Time/Round

NAME	RX	Load/Scale	Time/Round

NAME	RX	Load/Scale	Time/Round

NAME	RX	Load/Scale	Time/Round

BENCHMARK WORKOUT LOG

Load/Scale	Time/Round	Load/Scale	Time/Round	Load/Scale	Time/Round

Load/Scale	Time/Round	Load/Scale	Time/Round	Load/Scale	Time/Round

Load/Scale	Time/Round	Load/Scale	Time/Round	Load/Scale	Time/Round

Load/Scale	Time/Round	Load/Scale	Time/Round	Load/Scale	Time/Round

PERSONAL RECORD TRACKING

Deadlift						

Back Squat						

Press						

Bench Press						

Snatch						

Clean & Jerk						

1000m Row						

1 Mile Run						

PERSONAL RECORD TRACKING

NOTES

www.ingramcontent.com/pod-product-compliance
Lightning Source LLC
Chambersburg PA
CBHW060307290526
45789CB00001B/436